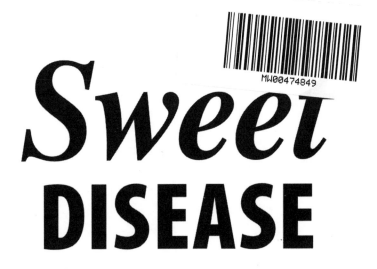

Sweet
DISEASE

What Sugar and Artificial Sweeteners are Doing to Your Health

By Brian Clement, Ph.D., NMD., L.N.
Foreword by Gary Null, Ph.D.

HIPP●CRATES
HEALTH INSTITUTE

Library of Congress Cataloging-in-Publication Data
is available from the Library of Congress.

ISBN-13: 978-1-4675-8056-4 (Paperback)
ISBN-10: 1-4675-8056-2 (Paperback)

© 2015 Brian R. Clement, PhD

Publisher: Hippocrates Health Institute
          1443 Palmdale Court
          West Palm Beach, FL 33411

Cover design by Larissa Hise Henoch
Inside design and formatting by Lawna Patterson Oldfield

*To all of the sweet people
who have the sweet disease of sugar
addiction; may you liberate yourself from
the crutches of this formidable,
disabling substance.*

*RECOMMENDED
DAILY SUGAR
CONSUMPTION
Women = 25 grams
men = 30 grams*

Table of Contents

Disclaimer: *The information in this book is presented for educational purposes only. It is not intended to be a substitute for the medical advice of your
health care professional. The state of Florida does not license Naturopathic
Medicine nor does the author practice these methods.*

Foreword
by Gary Null, PhD.

Nearly a century ago, the tobacco industry initiated a brilliant campaign of deception against the American people and the worldwide public. They were able to enlist the American Medical Association and its journal to run ads suggesting that cigarette smoking was in fact good for you, stating it would soothe your throat and calm your nerves. Big Tobacco's propaganda had infiltrated society to such an extent that even the majority of physicians smoked cigarettes.

For fifty years the tobacco industry's disinformation campaign was wildly successful. Tens of millions of Americans from my parents' generation smoked one to three packs a day from the 1920s to the 1970s. I grew up in a home where everyone smoked, as did my aunts and uncles. It would not be until the 1970s that the public was informed about the connection between cigarettes and damaging health consequences like emphysema and cancer. The insidious nature of Big Tobacco was revealed further in 1996 when Jeffrey Wigand, a tobacco company insider, went public with claims that industry executives intended to get consumers hooked on nicotine, and that these corporate leaders were well aware of the dangerous health effects that came with cigarette additives. By then it was too late to help my father, mother and brother, all of whom were heavy smokers and suffered from cancer. All told, tens of millions of people were injured or died from cigarettes. The truth finally came out and today there are label warnings from the Surgeon General on the health dangers of cigarette smoking and public awareness about the issue.

Today we witness the sugar industry's attempts to dismiss and discredit a substantial body of research showing the devastating effects of sugar on our wellbeing. In his new book, *Sweet Disease*, Brian Clement has come forward with the most important text on the dangers of sugar since William Duffy's *Sugar Blues* was published in 1975. As a lifelong advocate and educator who has helped countless individuals find greater vitality through healing diets high in raw foods and juices, Brian is eminently qualified to comment on the impact of sugar on health.

In *Sweet Disease*, Brian provides a comprehensive and authoritative look at the latest scientific evidence demonstrating how sugar takes a toll on so many areas of our health.

His exhaustive research paints a sobering picture of the link between America's addiction to sugar and our national epidemics of cancer, heart disease, diabetes, obesity, cognitive illness and other ailments. If people followed the advice in this book, I personally believe that we could be saving millions of lives and greatly reduce the suffering of tens of millions of people dealing with obesity and chronic degenerative disease.

This book is a timely reminder of the importance of making conscious choices about the foods we eat. Brian's work will undoubtedly help change the tide of worldwide opinion so that like tobacco, sugar will come to be widely known as the hazadous substance it truly is. This is a must read for those who care about living a longer and healthier life.

Gary Null, PhD.

Introduction:
An Unsweet Story, an Unhappy Ending

F ew people today realize it, or choose to think about it while consuming sugar in all its various forms, but 'white gold,' as British colonialists called the substance, was the primary driving force behind the introduction of slavery to the 'new world' in the 16th century. That remained true for 200 years until cotton and tobacco began to heavily target slave labor.

Millions of Africans were enslaved and then transported to sugar cane plantations throughout the Caribbean and South America where they were, quite literally, worked to death to produce a sweet-tasting product for the dietary pleasure of Europeans.

Slavery, as it was once practiced, may no longer be directly connected to the sugar trade, at least in our own century, yet a form of human bondage still links our species to the sugars that flow into human mouths from sugar cane and sugar beets. That bondage or yoke around our necks, the persistent and hard to eradicate slavery of body, mind and spirit, is a nasty addiction to sugar.

You may not want to believe it, you may choose to ignore it, but *sugar is more addictive than cocaine.* That's not me trying to exaggerate its evils. That's not me trying to sell books. That's a fact firmly rooted in science, as you will discover later in this book.

Sugar is tantamount to a drug and the addiction to it produces much more widespread illness and disease in humans than any other legal or even illegal drug, with the possible exception of tobacco.

Profiting richly from this addiction, while covering up its pernicious health repercussions and otherwise doing everything in their power to keep this addiction's tenacious hold in place over humans of all ages, is a sweetener industry more powerful than the tobacco industry had been at its zenith.

With hundreds of millions of dollars spent on campaign donations to politicians to pump up government subsidies and ward off regulation, and much more spent for propaganda extolling sugar usage and downplaying how it triggers disease and death, worldwide sweetener growers and producers, refiners, processed food manufacturers and fellow profit travelers constitute a clear and present danger to human health.

To spread the word about sugar and its associated cousins- the artificial sweeteners created and promoted as 'healthy' substitutes—I researched and wrote this book placing an emphasis on the most current medical science research revealing how a wide range of maladies from cancer to heart disease and neurological degeneration can be traced back to sweetener usage.

Sugar Purveyors Are Ruthless Drug Pushers

Of more than 85,000 processed food products sold on U.S. supermarket shelves today, at least 75% of them contain added sweeteners in one form or another. This number is consistent with most developed countries.

Corn syrup is the most common among these sweeteners, followed closely by sorghum, cane sugar and high-fructose corn syrup. Certain categories of foods are almost entirely dominated by individual sweeteners and combinations of sweeteners—for example, 95% of all cakes, cookies, pies, granola bars, protein bars, energy bars, cereals, and soda beverages contain high levels of added sweeteners.[1]

Don't be fooled by the labels 'healthy' and 'natural' because many of the products carrying such seductive words also

contain added sugars. You need to carefully read the ingredient labels. Even then, you must be a well-informed consumer
to identify the added sugars because they appear under 61
different names (see Chart One) ranging from dextrose and
maltose to rice syrup and barley malt. Nor will nutrition
labels on products give you the daily reference value for these
added sugars, as they do for fats and salt, since the U.S. Food
and Drug Administration doesn't require added sugars to be
estimated under its current labeling guidelines.

What sets unnatural sugars apart from natural sugar
sources? Two scientists, James DiNicolantonio of Saint
Luke's Mid America Heart Institute and Sean Lucan of the
Albert Einstein College of Medicine, explain how and what:
"Whereas natural sugar sources like whole fruits and vegetables are generally not very concentrated because the sweetness is buffered by water, fiber and other constituents, modern
industrial sugar sources are unnaturally potent and quickly
provide a big hit. Natural whole foods like beets are stripped
of their water, fiber, vitamins, minerals and other beneficial
components to produce purified sweetness. All that's left are
pure, white, sugar crystals. A comparison to drugs would not
be misplaced here. Similar refinement processes transform
other plants like poppies and coca into heroin and cocaine."[2]

How much added sweetener to our diets is too much? In
my view, any amount of added sugars is too much for the
human body to bear over the course of a lifetime. Medical

and nutritional advisory organizations are gradually catching up to this point of view.

Whereas the World Health Organization (WHO), for example, didn't address sugar as a profound health threat a decade ago, it now recommends limiting daily sugar consumption to 25 grams for women and 38 grams for men. This recommendation duplicates what The American Heart Association established as dietary guidelines. Still more support for that standard came in February 2015, when the Dietary Guidelines Advisory Committee, which every five years sends recommendations to the U.S. Department of Agriculture and the U.S. Department of Health and Human Services for shaping the nation's public school lunch programs, finally came around to identifying added sugars as a major health problem in need of addressing with cutbacks in consumption.[3]

The average U.S. citizen absorbs 82 grams of sugar a day from all sources, more than three times what WHO recommends for women and more than twice what it has set as a standard for men. If you extrapolate that daily consumption out over the course of a year, it comes to more than 66 pounds of added sugars for every person in the nation. These numbers are either identical, or close to that of all developed countries.[4]

My strong belief is that these estimates of added sugar in the average diet are way too conservative. Dr. Sanjay Gupta, the medical expert for CNN, voiced the same opinion, and in a March 2015 report estimated that the average American consumes *140 pounds of sugar a year*.[5]

To illustrate what I mean about sugars hiding everywhere in the typical diet, just a single 12-ounce soda contains 46 grams of added sugar. That's more than half of the estimated daily consumption of sugars in the mainstream American's diet. Think about how many people, particularly children and teens, drink two or more sodas or energy drinks daily.

Add to that the added sugars in everything from pasta sauce (12 grams in a half-cup) and ketchup (4 grams per tablespoon) to sweet salad dressings like raspberry vinaigrette (7 grams for every small serving) and such foods as yogurt (29 grams in a single serving) and bran cereal (20 grams per serving) and we're talking about a daily sugar intake *at least twice or three times* what medical associations, government agencies and nutritional authorities would have us believe.

We haven't even factored in the other major indirect source of sugars in the human body—refined carbohydrate products, which convert to sugar once absorbed. These foods include everything from bread and pasta to rice and related products. According to the U.S. Department of Agriculture, North Americans consume at least 200 pounds of grain products each year. That level of consumption raises the overall sugar ingested to nearly 400 pounds annually, so it's no wonder that the ideal metabolic conditions for cancer cells gets created in the human body.

A Sweet Disease Cover-up

Health problems and diseases linked to sugar consumption are legion and growing in number as research focuses on the disruptive power that sugar exercises over specific parts of the human chemistry and anatomy.

Many of these health maladies, such as cancer, heart disease, diabetes, and neurological diseases, are covered in detail with medical study verification elsewhere in the pages of this book. Other conditions triggered by sugar intake may surprise you even more than the lineup of usual suspects.

Consider these examples:

Did you know that your dietary sugar intake is a risk factor for the *development of cataracts*? Studies beginning in 2003 found a link between sugar and degeneration of the eyes resulting in cataracts.[6] *CATARACTS and sugar & salt consumption*

Did you ever consider that your sugar consumption, especially if you are a woman, is a risk factor for *depression*? More than 1,000 women aged 20 to 93 were studied to determine whether their sugar intake was connected to mental disorders, particularly depression. There was little doubt that such a link exists.[7]

Did you realize that your sugar habits help to determine whether you will contract *kidney disease*? Using a medical database of nearly 10,000 people 20 years of age and older, along with information on dietary habits, it was found that sugary soda consumption, by itself without even factoring in all of the other added dietary sugar sources, is associated with kidney disease.[8]

Taking not just a page but an entire chapter from the tobacco industry and its sordid history of lies and manipulations, the sugar industry, in all its various trade group and corporate forms, continues to employ the same tactics of spreading misinformation about the health dangers as Big Tobacco did. Meanwhile, it buys special treatment from public officials to protect sugar production and keep sugar consumption high.

For Halloween in 2010, The Sugar Association, a trade group that represents sugar cane and sugar beet producers and refiners, distributed 'fact sheets' for parents of trick or treating kids, claiming "sugar doesn't cause obesity" and "sugar adds to the quality of children's diets." To further reassure parents that eating candy is good for their kids, other 'fact sheets' issued by the group declared: "every major review of the scientific literature exonerates sugar as the cause of any disease, including obesity."[9]

These outright falsehoods might be simply laughable if they were isolated examples. But this type of propaganda is a common refrain heard from industries dependent on profits from the sale of sweeteners. For instance, still another food and beverage industry funded group, The International Food Information Council Foundation, posted a 2012 webpage stating: "to date, there is no conclusive evidence of a causative effect of sugars on chronic diseases."[10]

As might be expected, individual corporations that peddle sugars in their products also toe the sugar industry propaganda line by periodically jumping on the misinformation bandwagon. Here is what that purveyor of sugary cereals, the General Mills Corporation, alleged in a 2013 public statement: "sugar intake has not been shown to be directly associated with obesity or any chronic disease or health condition except dental caries."[11]

It's no wonder that a large segment of consumers find themselves confused about how much sugar is too much sugar before human health is seriously undermined. The same can be said, unfortunately, for many public officials who wield the power to keep consumers better informed about the health dangers of 'white gold' and its many sweet fellow travelers birthed in chemical laboratories.

Trying to Keep You
Fat, Ignorant, and Addicted

Taken together the sugar industry's "lobbying dollars, political contributions to lawmakers, and influence on rule making at federal agencies have all contributed to a lack of effective federal and state policies that would address the public health concerns of sugar consumption," concluded a report from policy analysts and scientists at the Center for Science and Democracy. "Decision makers seeking to enact such policies

have faced uphill battles, as sugar interests, through a combined force of these tactics, have swayed our public policies
on food, nutrition, and health."[12]

Even more in-depth examinations of how the sugar industry manipulates public policy, science, and public attitudes,
while siphoning off tax money as subsidies to prop up sugar
prices, can be found in the Union of Concern Scientists report,
*Sugar-coating Science: How the Food Industry Misleads Con-
sumers on Sugar.* You can also find detailed information in
the Marian Nestle book, *Food politics: How the food industry
influences nutrition and health.*

No examination of sweeteners and health would be com-
plete without weighing the effects of high fructose corn syrup
(HFCS), a sugar substitute made from corn starch that also
benefits from taxpayer subsidies that prop up corn prices. As
HFCS became a cheaper alternative to sugar for use in many
processed foods, from 1970 to 2000, according to the Center
for Science and Democracy, the production of HFCS par-
alleled the rise in obesity rates in the U.S. Author Michael
Pollard has laid out this correlation persuasively in the *New
York Times* and elsewhere.

Though HFCS manufacturers may be in competition with
sugar for consumer dollars, HFCS producers and product
packagers actually employ many of the same under handed
tactics as the sugar industry in promoting this corn-based
sweetener. One reason could be that HFCS triggers many of
the same or similar health problems sugar is known to trigger

or make worse, which inspires the HFCS interests and their lobby arms to use four manipulative strategies to disarm critics, as perfected by sugar interests:

- To ignore the science showing health hazards from their products using HFCS by emphasizing what science still doesn't know with certainty.

- By repeating false and misleading claims about the safety of HFCS, this industry tries to keep the public and policymakers confused.

- Scientific claims for HFCS safety are manufactured by the HFCS industry paying scientists to come up with findings that meet industry approval.

- Other claims supporting HFCS, none of which were published in respectable peer-reviewed science journals, are circulated and widely published in the industry trade journals.[13]

Coca-Cola is a good, healthy snack for people to have, according to 'nutritionists' and 'dietitians' hired by that corporation to spread such silliness. This misinformation campaign occurred in February 2015 for American Heart Month and consisted of newspaper columns and 1,000 online nutrition site and blog postings extolling the virtues of drinking this particular soda.

So exactly how is a can of Coca-Cola, chock full of high fructose corn syrup, a health drink? The so-called 'experts' hired to make health claims weren't very specific in their media campaign, except to claim they had scientific evidence that soda wasn't a risk to heart health and it wasn't responsible for the obesity epidemic.

One of these mercenary dietitians on the Coca-Cola payroll, Robyn Flipse, told Associated Press that she doesn't drink sodas herself, but she is willing to urge others to drink it in return for Coca-Cola payments. She confessed that any time she sees articles or studies blaming sugary drinks for health problems, she contacts the public relations agencies for the criticized product and asks, "Do you want me to do something about that?"[14]

Flipse's dozens of corporate clients range from Coca-Cola and the American Beverage Association to Splenda the sweetener company, from Kraft and Kellogg's to Tyson Foods. Here is how she describes her services for food corporations on her personal website: "Do you need a Nutrition Consultant who is able to develop, evaluate, and execute your new product ideas and marketing objectives? Are you looking for a Spokesperson who can deliver your food, nutrition and health messages accurately and articulately? Can you use a food, nutrition and health Author who gets the facts right and delivers the copy for your target audience within budget and on time? Then look no further because Robyn Flipse can do it all for you! She is a Registered Dietitian with 25 years of experience in corporate consulting and media relations who has her finger on the pulse of the ever evolving trends in food, nutrition, diet and health."[15]

One of the claims made by Coca-Cola and other soda manufacturers revolves around the notion that all sugars are created equal. In other words, liquid sugar, which is the biggest source of added sugar in your diet, is not much different from the sugars we absorb naturally from fruits.

This attempt to manipulate and capitalize on consumer ignorance about natural sugars was thoroughly debunked by independent nutrition and health scientists associated with the non-profit group, SugarScience, based at the University of California, San Francisco.[16]

"Research suggests that our bodies process liquid sugar differently than sugar in foods, especially those containing fiber," SugarScience researchers reported. "When we eat an apple, for example, we may be getting as many as 18 grams of sugar, but the sugar is 'packaged' with about one-fifth of our daily requirement of fiber. Because it takes our bodies a long time to digest that fiber, the apple's sugar is slowly released into our blood stream, giving us a sustained source of energy. But when we drink the same amount of sugar in sugary drinks, it doesn't include that fiber. As a result, the journey from liquid sugar to blood sugar happens quickly, delivering more sugar to the body's vital organs than they can handle. Over time, that can overload the pancreas and liver, leading to serious diseases like diabetes, heart disease and liver disease."[17]

Raise the Alarm about Added Sugars

Not just as a nation, not just as a culture or society, do we need to confront the health implications of consuming added sugars. We must confront our addiction to these substances as a *species*, the human species, because the effects of sweet poison will shape the future of generations to come, starting in the womb.

Most human beings no longer consider added sugars in their diet as a condiment to be consumed only periodically; they accept added sugars as a dietary staple. This is a habit that must be broken. Wider education about the health dangers is an essential start down that road.

"As pediatricians, we had evidence of the connection between sugar and diabetes, heart disease and liver disease for years, but we haven't had this level of definitive scientific evidence to back up our concerns," observed Dr. Robert Lustig, a pediatric endocrinologist and a member of the SugarScience team at the University of California, San Francisco. That medical science team reviewed more than 8,000 published scientific papers about the health dangers of sweetener consumption with the aim of taking this information out of medical journals and disseminating it in accessible form to the public so healthy choices can be made.

SugarScience released a statement in November 2014 noting that with "the overwhelming negative findings associated with sugar consumption, the good news is that the knowledge

can empower people to change their habits. The most important step is understanding how much we eat, as well as where
in our diet that sugar comes from."[18]

Those who publicly challenge the soft drink and processed
foods industries often end up being targeted in smear and
slander campaigns. I have seen this firsthand as trolls sur-
face on the Internet attacking me and the Hippocrates Health
Institute each time I have spoken out about the sugar and
high fructose corn syrup menace to public health. If anything,
these attacks have only served to embolden me in speaking
the truth.

My goal with this book, *Sweet Disease*, is to further advance
the accessibility and availability of the body of science knowledge about sweeteners so that eventually no one has an excuse
to remain uninformed about what these toxic substances are
doing to human health.

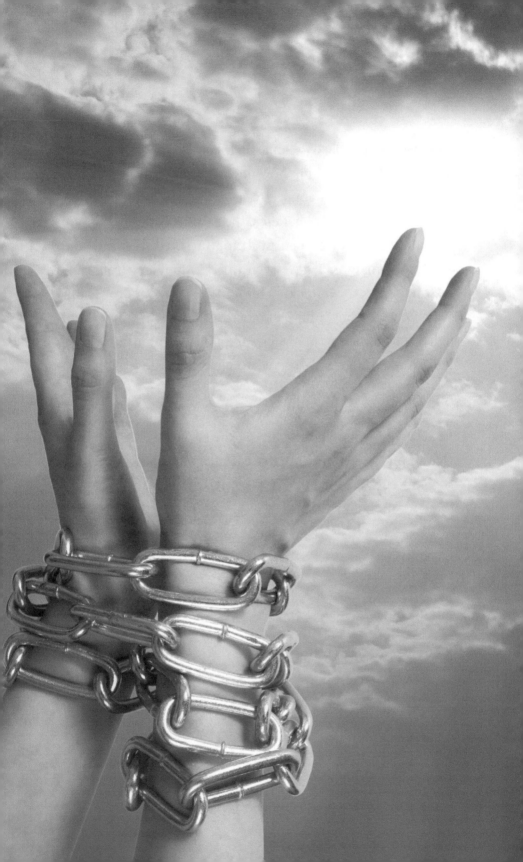

Chapter One

Sugar's Sordid Timeline History

S ugar is an umbrella term for sweetness in its many forms—cane sugar, beet sugar, honey, molasses, fruit juice concentrate, maple syrup, high-fructose corn syrup, agave nectar, among the many naturally-occurring and synthetically-derived sweeteners known to humans. In early recorded history it was mostly a sweetener experience dominated by sugar cane and honey, and that is where our story begins.

8,000 BC—It is conjectured that sugar cane was first domesticated in New Guinea and its cultivation then spread to Southeast Asia, China, and then beyond.[20, 28]

2,400 BC—Earliest evidence of beekeeping in hives to collect honey for honey cakes found at a religious temple near present day Cairo, Egypt.[19, 35]

350 AD—Sugarcane growers in India discover and master how to crystallize sugar using a boiling process of refining cane juice.[32]

11th Century—British and French Christian crusaders encounter sugar from sugar cane grown by Arabs and bring back this 'new spice' to their own lands where it becomes an expensive delicacy for the rich and nobility.[20, 28]

1319—A kilo of sugar (known as 'white gold') goes for two shillings a pound in London, the equivalent of about $50 a pound in current dollars, keeping it a luxury item that few people below the richest class will experience in a lifetime.[20, 28]

1493—On his second voyage to the 'new' world of the Americas, Christopher Columbus brings along sugar cane plant seedlings for planting in the Caribbean islands of Hispaniola, where the warm climate is conducive for growth of the plant, giving rise to the sugar cane industry.[20, 28]

16th Century—Native Americans are enslaved by Europeans throughout the Caribbean islands, particularly Barbados and Jamaica, and in Central and South America, as labor to harvest sugar cane. When their numbers become depleted by disease and harsh working conditions, African slaves are shipped in to take their place in the fields and processing operations. Millions will die in the sugar cane fields from the brutal labor, lack of medical care, or in attempting to escape imprisonment.[20, 34, 37]

1700—An average person in Britain consumes four pounds of sugar a year; that amount will gradually increase as the price of sugar falls due to overproduction in the Americas, making it affordable for the middle class and poor.[34, 37]

1747—Sugar beets are identified as a new source of commercial sugar. This new source further drives down world prices and makes sugar more affordable to generations of lower and middle class people never exposed to it before. Sugar is being added to jams, candy, tea, coffee, and many other food items.[28]

1800—A French medical student identifies the first series of patients with Rheumatoid Arthritis, a condition characterized by the body's own immune system attacking joint linings and cartilage. Two centuries later medical research will link sugar consumption as a cause of Rheumatoid Arthritis.[29, 38]

1807—By the time Britain bans slave trading in this year, at least six million African slaves have been incarcerated on sugar cane plantations.[34, 37]

1870—The average resident of Britain consumes 47 pounds of sugar a year.[20, 34, 37]

1880—Cheaper sugar beets now replace sugar cane as the principal sugar source for Europeans.[28]

1890—Indentured servants now eclipse slaves as the primary work force worldwide growing and processing sugar. An estimated 450,000 indentured servants, most serving ten years or more in servitude, are moved around the world, most to Fiji, Hawaii, and Australia. Once indentured servitude ends in the early 20th Century, sugar production remains an industry characterized by meager wages and workers living in harsh working conditions and extreme poverty.[34]

1900—The average Briton now eats about 100 pounds of sugar annually; the average American consumes 40 pounds.[37]

1906—A German physician, Dr. Alzheimer, first identifies a form of dementia characterized by dramatic shrinkage in brain nerve cells. By the end of the 20th century, an estimated 5 million Americans a year will be diagnosed with Alzheimer's disease.[30]

1910—A medical explanation emerges in the U.S. for the rising rates of diabetes: the pancreas of a diabetes patient was unable to produce what {is} termed "insulin," a chemical the body uses to break down sugar. Thus, excess sugar ended up in the urine.[25, 27]

1962—An estimated 13% of American adults meet the criteria for obesity.[21]

1967—A Japanese scientist invents a cost-effective industrial process for using enzymes to convert glucose in cornstarch to fructose. High Fructose Corn Syrup derived from corn becomes a cheap alternative sweetener to sugar.[28]

1975—In the U.S. 400 new cases of cancer occur for every 100,000 people.[23, 24]

1984—Soft drink manufacturers such as Pepsi and Coca-Cola switch from sugar to the cheaper high-fructose corn syrup in U.S. production facilities.[35]

1992—Cancer rates have climbed to 510 new cases for every 100,000 people in the U.S.[23, 24]

1997—An estimated 19.4% of U.S. adults meet criteria for obesity.[21]

2004—Obesity now affects 24.5% of U.S. adults.[21]

2005—Each U.S. citizen eats about 100 pounds of added sugars each year, up from about 40 pounds in 1900.[33]

2008—An ordinary American now consumes 37.8 pounds of high-fructose corn syrup every year, mostly unknowingly because it is laced in thousands of processed food and drink products. It is considered one of the 'hidden' sweeteners because, like many sugars and artificial sweeteners, it uses numerous chemical aliases making it difficult to identify on food label ingredient lists.[21]

2008—The obesity rate for adult Americans reaches 32.2% of men and 35.5% of women. Obesity is considered a contributing factor to the deaths of nearly 400,000 Americans annually.[26]

2009—The American Heart Association issues health recommendations that women consume no more than six teaspoons per day of sugars and men consume no more than nine teaspoons a day. Generally both men and women consume three times that amount daily.[26]

2015—The Dietary Guidelines Advisory Committee, which meets every five years to issue dietary recommendations to the U.S. Department of Health and Human Services and the U.S. Department of Agriculture, advises for the first time that American consumers dramatically cut back on the amount of added sugars to 12 teaspoons a day, half of what Americans currently consume. Much of these added sugars are derived from consumption of juices, sodas and a wide range of sugary drinks.[35, 36]

(See References section at the end of the book for sources.)

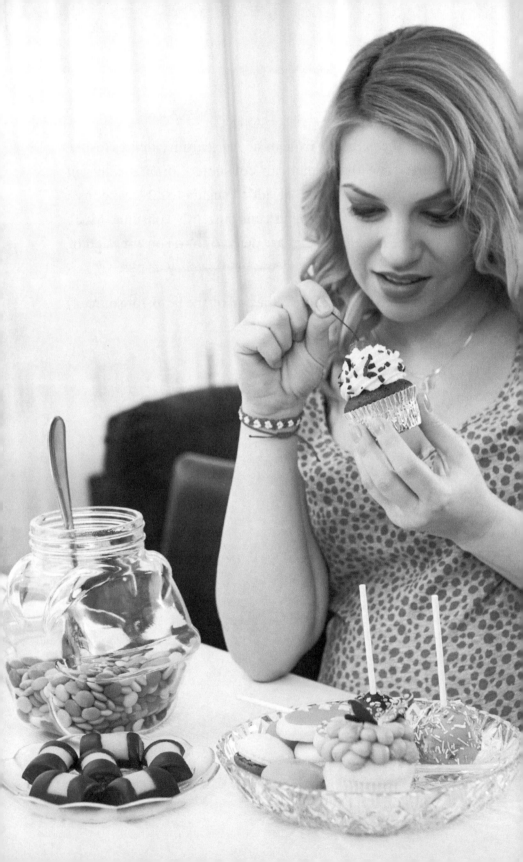

Chapter Two

Our Most Addictive Substance

For decades it's been a running joke among members of Alcoholic's Anonymous (AA) and Narcotic's Anonymous (NA)—'get off the drugs and alcohol and get on the sugar.'

At just about any AA or NA meeting anywhere in the world you will find in the back of the meeting room tables laden with donuts, candies, cookies and sugar in every imaginable form. It's the same scene at drug and alcohol rehabilitation centers where sodas, sugary juices, sugary snacks and energy drinks are distributed promiscuously to addicts who are unknowingly substituting one addiction for another.

Even the AA's 'Big Book' as it is known, the 12 Step bible written by AA's founder, urges addicts to eat candy when going sober because sugar is considered 'harmless' as a substitute for alcohol and drugs.

What happens to many, if not most, drug and alcohol addicts is they transfer their drug cravings into an addiction to sugar, a phenomenon now called 'transfer addicting.' The result is that many newly sober people put on extra weight and that added weight translates into Type 2 diabetes and a range of other health problems, as this book will demonstrate in coming chapters.

"Off the cocaine, onto the cupcakes," remarked Dr. Pamela Peeke, an assistant professor of medicine at the University of Maryland, in a 2014 interview with *The New York Times*. "Once off the drugs, the brain craves the rewards of Mint Milanos, Oreos, any sugar."

Convincing evidence that sugar has an addictive influence on the human brain's reward center, an effect more powerful than many addictive drugs, has come from medical science studies conducted over just the past few years.

A team of French scientists in 2007 did animal studies in which mammals were given a choice between intravenous cocaine or water sweetened with either saccharin or sucrose, a natural sugar. Most of the animals, 94% of them, preferred the sweet taste over their cocaine habit, no matter how much cocaine they were administered.

"Our findings clearly demonstrate that intense sweetness can surpass cocaine reward, even in drug-sensitized and addicted individuals," wrote the science team in a science journal article. "In most mammals, including humans, sweet receptors evolved in ancestral environments poor in sugars and are thus not adapted to high concentrations of sweet tastants. The supranormal stimulation of these receptors by sugar-rich diets, such as those now widely available in modern societies, would generate a supranormal reward signal in the brain, with the potential to override self-control mechanisms and thus to lead to addiction."[39]

Other research by Professor Bart Hoebel and scientists at the Princeton University Neuroscience Institute in 2008 documented how sugar releases the hormone dopamine in the brain and with repetition, or binge eating, this consumption results in sugar addiction. Over time neurochemical changes occur in the brain "that appear to mimic those produced by substances of abuse, including cocaine, morphine and nicotine," said Hoebel. "In certain models, sugar bingeing causes long-lasting effects in the brain and increases the inclination to take other drugs of abuse, such as alcohol."[40]

As further evidence of sugar's addictive power, when lab animals had their sugar supply taken away, the levels of dopamine in their brains dropped. As a result, these lab sugar addicts exhibited all of the classic signs of drug withdrawal seen in humans, such as anxiety, restlessness, fear and even teeth chattering. If sugar was reintroduced to their diet, these animals consumed sugar ravenously and in larger quantities than they ever had before, showing the relapse potential.

These study results should have been immediately embraced by the entire substance addictions treatment industry. Feeding addicts sugar is simply going to prime their brains for future relapse. It's no wonder that drug and alcohol addiction is so difficult to treat and relapse rates are so high.

As experiments with lab animals and sugar addiction became more sophisticated, so did the detail derived in explaining how sugar addicts the brain. Neuroscientists at Connecticut College place Oreo cookies, those crème-filled sugar products, on one side of the cage with injections of cocaine or morphine available on the other side. The animals gravitated to the cookies. When the research team measured the pleasure centers of the rat's brains, they noted clear evidence that Oreo cookies activated more neurons to control behavior than did either morphine or cocaine. Not only that, rats preferred to eat the cookies by breaking it open and eating the sugar-laden crème first, much as humans do, before eating the chocolate wafers surrounding it.[41]

Just to be sure that it is sugar and not fat that humans crave most, MRI scans have been done of human brains when milkshakes were consumed. When researchers took the sugar away from the milkshakes and left the milk fats, the brains didn't light up with glee nearly as much as they did when the sugar was back in the drink.

Once these and related study findings about sugar and addiction were replicated and confirmed, the floodgates of research opened up exploring the intricacies and implications of this relationship.

✓ "The model of sugar bingeing has been used successfully to elicit behavioral and neurochemical signs of dependence: indices of opiate-like withdrawal, increased intake after abstinence, cross-sensitization with drugs of abuse, and the repeated release of dopamine."[42]

✓ "It has been observed that the biological children of alcoholic parents, particularly alcoholic fathers, are at greater risk to have a strong sweet preference and may manifest in some with an eating disorder."[43]

✓ "Research has revealed that sugar and sweet reward can not only substitute to addictive drugs, like cocaine, but can even be more rewarding and attractive. At the neurobiological levels, the neural substrates of sugar and sweet reward appear to be more robust than those of cocaine possibly reflecting past selective evolutionary pressures for seeking and taking foods high in sugar and calories."[44]

This recent research provides the scientific proof for an idea that's been a cultural rumor since the 1960's and 1970's: sugar is a poison. The late Hollywood star Gloria Swanson crusaded on the theme that sugar consumption creates ill health until her death, and then her husband, William Dufty, continued the campaign with a 1975 book, *Sugar Blues*, in which he wrote: "the difference between sugar addiction and narcotic addiction is largely one of degree. After all, heroin is nothing but a chemical. They take the juice of the poppy and they refine it into opium and then they refine it to morphine and finally to heroin. Sugar is nothing but a chemical. They take the juice of the cane or the beet, and they refine it to molasses and then they refine it to brown sugar and finally to strange white crystals."

Still another cultural sign that aware people were waking up to the addictive potential of sugar before medical science did came in the 1955 movie, *The Man With the Golden Arm,* starring Frank Sinatra and Kim Novak. For those of you who don't remember or weren't born yet, Sinatra played a heroin addict who discovers he is also a sugar addict when he kicks the heroin addiction. In one famous scene after kicking heroin, Sinatra says:

"The most gorgeous day I ever saw. I got a craving from something sweet. You got anything sweet?"

"Sugar," said the Novak character.

"Gimme."

In response she pours a fountain of sugar into his cupped hands.

Sinatra licks the sugar and demands more.

"How can you?" says the Novak character, making a displeased face.

"I never felt this good in my life," says Sinatra, ravenously eating more sugar. "I feel like all the things inside me settled into place."

Other Hollywood films made the same or a similar point. In the 1962 movie, *The Days of Wine and Roses*, the alcoholic played by Jack Klugman revealed to his friend, played by Jack Lemmon, that he knew his wife was an alcoholic because of her obsession with eating chocolate candy.

Now that we know without scientific doubt and beyond mere cultural rumors that sugar triggers addiction, and that sugar is even more addictive than alcohol or cocaine, what should be done to warn consumers and to protect human health?

The public health policy implications of sugar being named an addictive drug were examined in a 2013 paper in the *Journal of Law and Medical Ethics*. "What was once a naturally occurring food ingredient is now a highly concentrated food additive. If foods containing artificially high levels of sugar are capable of triggering addictive behaviors, how should policy makers respond? What regulatory steps would be suitable and practical?"[45]

The obvious answer is for the U.S. Food and Drug Administration to declare added sugar in all its various forms to be a highly-addictive substance in need of regulation like any other addictive drug. As you can imagine, such a step will be fanatically resisted by the sugar and processed foods industries, just as Big Tobacco fought with its huge financial resources against the designation of nicotine as an addictive substance.

Breeding Sugars In and Nutrition Out

Over the centuries, genetic alterations in the domesticated fruits and plants were brought about by selection and the use of pollination practices, which produced ever sweeter hybrids. Human taste buds adapted as diets got sweeter, which further increased the desire for sweetness in the food supply.

This sweetness preference was a continually progressive process as new fruits were domesticated and the addictive potential of sugars was exploited. As a major plant breeding journal pointed out: "In the late Neolithic and Bronze Ages between 6000 and 3000 BCE, the ancient Mediterranean fruits (date, olive, grape, fig, sycamore fig, and pomegranate) were domesticated. Fruits such as citrus, banana, various pome fruits (apple, pear, quince, medlar) and stone fruits (almond, apricot, cherry, peach, and plum) were domesticated in Central and East Asia and reached the West in antiquity. A number of fruits and nuts were domesticated only in the 19th and 20th Centuries (blueberry, blackberry, pecan, and kiwifruit)."[46]

Increases in sweetness intensity, a direct result of selective breeding, has been documented as occurring in most fruits, though the more significant transformations have been seen in apples, pears, blueberries, strawberries, cherries, grapes, peaches and plums.[47]   ? WATERMELONS

Consider how corn in grocery stores got super sweet. A plant geneticist in 1959 developed a mutant strain of corn that was ten times sweeter than ordinary corn. He began selling the first hybrids in 1961 and since then, these super sugary varieties of corn dominated the market. "The sweetest varieties approach 40 percent sugar, bringing new meaning to the words 'candy corn,'" reported The New York Times in 2013. "We've reduced the nutrients and increased the sugar and starch content of hundreds of other fruits and vegetables."[48]

Along with these progressive increases in sugar content, plant breeders depleted the content of phyto-nutrients, the chemicals responsible for many of the healing qualities and disease prevention attributes that turn food into medicine for humans, by focusing on new varieties that resist fungus growth and plant diseases. These plant breeders simply don't seem to care that they have depleted the nutritional content and human health has suffered as a result.

The Tobacco and Sugar Connection

It's no longer a secret that cigarettes contain hundreds of chemical additives, many of them toxic, and many of them designed to enhance the effects of nicotine in the human body. What you may not know is that sugar is one of those additives.

Research conducted by the British group, Action on Smoking and Health, established by the Royal College of Physicians, delved into thousands of pages of internal tobacco company documents released as a result of consumer lawsuits and found the following:

✓ Sugar and other additives "are used to enhance the taste of tobacco smoke." The sugars react with added ammonia to help produce a milder tasting smoke.

✓ Sweeteners and chocolate are used to "help make cigarettes more palatable to children and first time users."

✓ Additives "such as cocoa may be used to dilate the airways allowing the smoke an easier and deeper passage into the lungs exposing the body to more nicotine."[49]

Adding sugar to tobacco serves another important function in the tobacco industry's attempt to manufacture nicotine dependence: "it enhances the addictive effects of nicotine," the British medical group discovered. The burning of sugars produces a chemical called acetaldehyde, which interacts with nicotine to produce a synergistic effect of heightened addiction potential.

"Senior Philip Morris scientist Victor J. DeNoble began research in the early eighties into the behavioural effects of nicotine and acetaldehyde in rats," the British scientists revealed. "He discovered that the two drugs worked synergistically to enhance the addictive nature of nicotine . . . Following this discovery DeNoble and his team were ordered to find the optimal ratio of the two compounds. According to DeNoble {in later public testimony} once the company had discovered the optimal ratio for addiction they increased the levels of sugar in Marlboro cigarettes to achieve the required increase in levels of acetaldehyde."

So there we have it. It's not just that the sugar industry uses the same marketing and political tactics as the tobacco industry to protect the market share profits for their addictive products. Nicotine and sugar are cut from the same cloth of addiction and work together in symbiotic ways to enslave humanity.

How Many Are Addicted?

At least 70% of all people in developed countries have a sugar addiction, estimated Dr. Fred Pescatore, the former medical director of the Atkins Center for Complementary Medicine in New York. His guess may be conservative.

Upwards of 90% of everyone in the U.S. alone are cer-
tifiable sugar addicts, claims Dr. Michael Lam, the medical
education director of the Academy of Anti-Aging Research.
He says that being addicted to sugar is now the norm.

Blame for sugar addiction being the norm, if we are to get
at the root of the problem, must go to those food scientists
working for food and beverage processors who have been paid
handsomely to create combinations of ingredients that stim-
ulate human dependence. Former head of the U.S. Food and
Drug Administration, Dr. David Kessler, revealed in his book
The End of Overeating how even synthetic opiates are being
added to heighten sensory effects and increase dependence.

Physicians Committee for Responsible Medicine founder
Dr. Neal Barnard describes their blame quite succinctly:
"They're trying to make the foods as seductive as possible. A
chocolate manufacturer spends endless hours and millions of
dollars trying to figure out the most seductive combination of
fat and sugar that triggers chocolate addiction and makes it
impossible to break it. Or a soda manufacturer has pushed up
serving sizes and made sure that addictive ingredients such as
sugar and caffeine are kept in the mix. They have made these
into addictive products to make money."[50]

As you will learn in the following chapters, addiction to
sugar triggers multiple human health problems and diseases
that cost consumers and wider society untold billions of dollars in medical bills. Continue reading. You will find the case
against sugar and its sweetener cousins to be overwhelming.

CHART 1: Sugars Hidden Under Pseudonyms on Food Labels

Processed food manufacturers do not like to advertise the fact that they are playing a deceptive game with your health by hiding added sugars on food product labels. They do this manipulation of public tastes using dozens of often contrived names for the substance—61 names altogether—which enable the corporations to ramp up the addictive sweetness power of their products to expand sales.

As a result of these 'hidden persuaders,' it's virtually impossible for you, the average consumer, to calculate or learn how much added sugar you are actually consuming with each product, unless you carry around this list of 61 sugar names all the time. Even then, an added impediment to your knowledge comes with the absence of any 'daily reference value' sugar information on labels, unlike fats and salt content which are required in the U.S. to be labeled according to daily reference values.

Just so you know, for future buying reference, here are the 61 sugar pseudonyms commonly used in processed foods sold in the U.S. and many other countries, listed alphabetically. Keep in mind that combinations of these sugars are often used in supermarket products.

Agave nectar	Coconut palm sugar
Barbados sugar	Coconut sugar
Barley malt	Confectioner's sugar
Barley malt syrup	Corn sweetener
Beet sugar	Corn syrup
Brown sugar	Corn syrup solids
Buttered syrup	Date sugar
Cane Juice	Dehydrated cane juice
Cane juice crystals	Demerara sugar
Cane sugar	Dextrin
Caramel	Dextrose
Carob syrup	Evaporated cane juice
Castor sugar	Free-flowing brown sugars

Fructose	Maltodextrin
Fruit juice	Maltol
Fruit juice concentrate	Maltose
Glucose	Mannose
Glucose solids	Maple syrup
Golden sugar	Molasses
Golden syrup	Muscovado
Grape sugar	Palm sugar
High-Fructose Corn Syrup (HFCS)	Panocha
Honey	Powdered sugar
Icing sugar	Raw sugar
Invert sugar	Refiner's syrup
Malt syrup	Rice syrup

Saccharose	Syrup
Sorghum syrup	Treacle
Sucrose	Turbinado sugar
Sugar (granulated)	Yellow sugar
Sweet sorghum	

(From: *Sugar Science*, University of California, San Francisco. *www.sugarscience.org*)

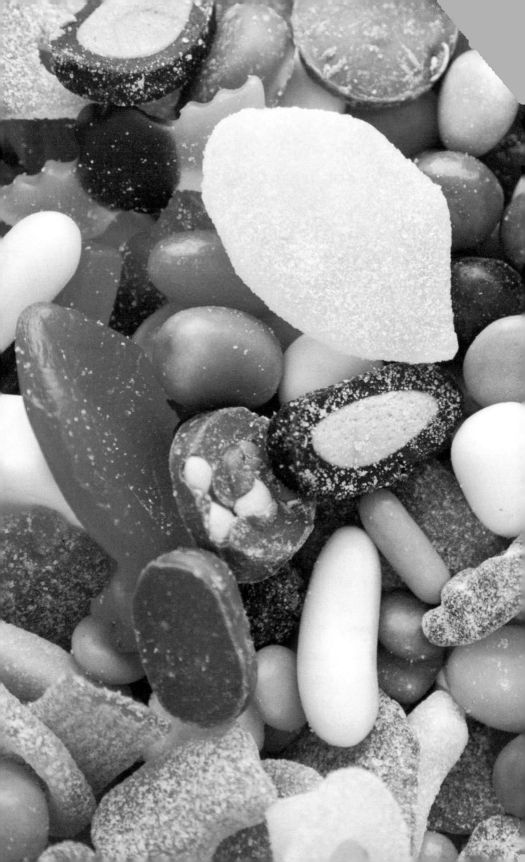

CHART TWO: Sweetener Families
from Nature & Laboratories

? complex sugars
? sources
? grams!!
? other

Simple sugars are sucrose, glucose, and fructose, all found naturally in whole foods and often added to processed foods to intensify sweetness.

Sucrose—commonly known as table sugar, in nature it is derived in its highest concentrations from red beets and sugar cane. Once consumed, it separates in the human body into units of fructose and glucose. Glucose is used as the body's primary energy source.

? raisins

Fructose—commonly called fruit sugar, found in all dried fruit and comes naturally highest in grapes. It is only metabolized in the human liver and behaves like a fat in the body. Medical study data show it to be a contributory to premature aging and a range of diseases.

? fatty
belly
Fat
hips

High Fructose Corn Syrup (HFCS)—a form of liquid sugar, highly concentrated, artificially refined from corn starch. Three types of HFCS are produced when glucose molecules are converted into fructose, each of the three with a different concentration of fructose and glucose. The first type of HFCS is used in soft drinks as a sweetener; the other two types appear most often in processed foods such as baked goods. Most corn used to manufacture HFCS is genetically modified.

*? SPLENDA
* SWEET & LOW*

Artificial sweeteners—four in particular stand out for their documented dangers to health: **Aspartame, Acesulfame-K, Sucralose,** and **Saccharin.**

Aspartame contains the chemicals phenylalanine, aspartic acid and methanol, which have been shown to directly affect brain and central nervous system functions in humans; side effects from its use may include, but are not limited to, memory loss, headaches, neurological disorders, irritable bowel syndrome, fibromyalgia, arthritis, visions problems and weight gain.

Acesulfame-K contains a potassium salt with methylene chloride, an identified carcinogen; side effects from its use include liver and kidney impairment, headaches, nausea, mood disorders, and possible cancers.

Sucralose is created by chlorinating sugar, whose chemical structure resembles that of the banned pesticide, DDT. Side effects from its use include inflammation, head and muscle aches, stomach cramps and bladder problems. Studies have found that it negatively impacts liver and kidney function.

Saccharin is sulfa-based with benzoic sulfimide as the primary ingredient. Anyone with a sulfa allergy may experience nausea, diarrhea and other symptoms from its use. Conflicting study evidence shows a possible link to bladder cancer. It has also been considered a detriment to health for decades.

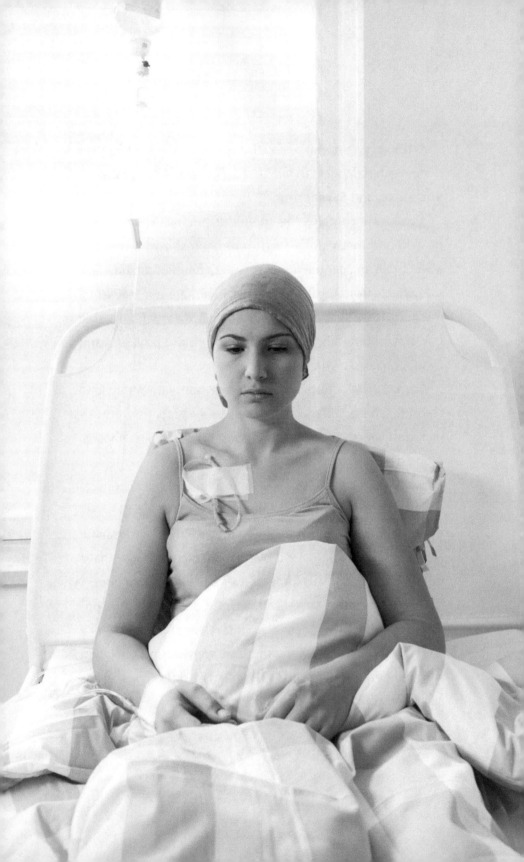

Chapter Three

Cancer Cells Get Addicted to Sugar, Too

I t's not only a sign of how far we've come but how far we've yet to go!

Most cancer research and treatment centers 'educated' their patients about sugar consumption and cancer as recently as 2012 using this sort of misguided language: "Research shows that eating sugar doesn't necessarily lead to cancer. It's what sugar does to your waistline that can lead to cancer…Should you avoid sugar? Our expert says no." This was from the MD Anderson Cancer Center, posted on their website in November 2012.[51]

As medical science has discovered—and as we at Hippocrates Health Institute have been warning for decades—this conventional medical advice and 'wisdom' about sugar and its relationship to cancer is just plain WRONG!

Since at least 1923 scientists have known that cancer tumor cells use much more glucose than do normal cells. The significance of this finding was mostly overlooked during the subsequent decades as the war on cancer consumed billions of dollars in research funding from the federal government and private sources.

Beginning in 1993 and beyond, medical science studies began popping up in various medical journals showing the effects of the Big Three Sweeteners—glucose, sucrose and fructose—in accelerating the progression of colon cancer in laboratory animals. Epidemiological studies done with large groups of human subjects followed over many years detected a similar pattern of correlations between sugar consumption and cancer risk.

Then, in 2009, a further breakthrough came when a team of researchers at the Huntsman Cancer Institute, University of Utah, uncovered convincing evidence of a direct link showing how sugar actually 'feeds' cancer tumors. Though both glucose (sugar) and glutamine (an amino acid) are essential for normal cell development as well as cancer cell growth, these had been thought to be independent processes. But this study showed their interdependence: when glutamine availability to the cell ceased, so did glucose utilization by the cell, which in

w/ CANCER = NO FRUIT

turn halted cancer cell growth. These researchers documented that depriving cancer cells of sugar via glucose was one way to arrest and treat cancer growth. These study findings were subsequently published in the *Proceedings of the National Academy of Sciences.*[52]

Fructose drew similar attention and a damning rebuke in 2011 when researchers at the University of California's Geffen School of Medicine reported that "recent observations indicate that cancer cells readily utilize fructose to support proliferation and dietary fructose can promote cancer growth by a variety of mechanisms, including altered cellular metabolism, increased reactive oxygen species, DNA damage and inflammation." Cancer cells were found to utilize fructose in similar but different ways than refined sugars, but lethal nonetheless.[53]

This fructose consumption link to cancer was further elaborated on in a 2012 study that explained why fructose "promotes a more aggressive cancer," particularly pancreatic and small intestinal cancers. A process called glycolysis is the major pathway stimulating cancer growth and "fructose provides an alternative carbon source for glycolysis."[54]

Still more evidence for sugar's cancer link, further nailing down exactly how sugar molecules cause cancer cell growth, came in 2013 from the University of Copenhagen where scientists discovered "that immature sugar molecules in the form of truncated 0-glycans aid growth properties of cancer cells." This interaction results in the cancer spreading more aggressively. "Our finding guides our entire field of research towards new ways to proceed in the battle against cancer," said co-author of the study, Catharina Steentoft, with the Department of Cellular and Molecular Medicine, University of Copenhagen, Denmark.

To compound the toxic effects of consuming sugar, if you eat meat and dairy products you are even more of a cancer statistic waiting to happen. As a cancer and other health malady trigger, the evidence for toxic synergies—the molecular interactions that occur between sugars, fats and meats—has emerged in the study literature as a threat that any sane person should take into consideration.

Here is an example of one such study:

"We prospectively evaluated the relation between dietary patterns and risk among 72,113 women who were followed up from 1984 to 2002. A Western pattern diet reflected high intakes of red meat, processed meat, refined grains, French fries, and **sweets/desserts**, was associated with a higher risk of mortality from cardiovascular disease (22% higher), cancer (16% higher) and all causes (21%) than a prudent diet with high intakes of vegetables."[55]

One scientist at the forefront of showing how sugars can trigger and accelerate cancerous tumor growths is Thomas N. Seyfried, Ph.D., a Yale University and Boston College expert on the biochemistry of cancer. He wrote a pioneering 2012 book, *Cancer as a Metabolic Disease: On the Origin, Management, and Prevention of Cancer.*

In this book, Seyfried confidently made this declaration: "glucose accelerates tumor growth."

Based on numerous studies with both lab animals and human brain cancer patients, Seyfried concluded that "the higher the glucose level {as measured in blood} the faster is the cancer growth. As glucose levels fall, tumor size (weight) and growth rate falls."

This scientist directly challenges the reigning orthodoxy in the field of oncology with his well-supported work showing that elimination of dietary sugars and the overall reductions in calorie intake fight cancer much more effectively than toxic drugs.

He calls "the dependence of tumor cells on glucose and glutamine for survival as the 'Achilles heel' of cancer," a vulnerability that can be exploited using dietary energy reduction, otherwise known as calorie restriction or fasting.

"In contrast to most conventional cancer therapies, which cause tissue necrosis and inflammation, metabolic therapies involving reduced calorie intake primarily kill tumor cells through apoptotic cell death," wrote Seyfried. "Is it better to kill tumor cells using toxic drugs, as is currently done in the oncology field, or is it better to kill tumor cells using a nontoxic metabolic therapy DER (dietary energy reduction)? I favor the latter approach."

With the abundance of medical science evidence cited above, why would any thinking person continue soaking his/her innards with sugars, particularly after receiving a cancer diagnosis? Why won't oncologists warn their patients about the dangers of continuing to consume sugar in any form?

It can only be due to sugar addiction combined with a prevailing stubborn ignorance of the dangers.

In 2013, the estimated new cancer cases diagnosed reached 1.6 million in the U.S. alone, with nearly 600,000 annual deaths from the various forms of cancer.[56]

Four of the most common and deadly types of cancer – breast, colon, endometrial and pancreatic—also happen to be the cancers where the most documentation exists to show a direct link with sugar consumption.

Let's take a closer look at that evidence.

Strongest Cancer/ Sugar Links: Breast; Colon; Endometrial; Pancreatic.

Significant Breast Cancer Studies:

"We investigated the association between breast cancer and high intake of sweets in a population-based case-control study of 1,434 cases and 1,440 controls from Long Island, NY. Consumption of a food grouping that included dessert foods, sweet beverages, and added sugars was positively associated with breast cancer risk. These results are consistent with other studies that implicate insulin-related factors in breast carcinogenesis."

Consumption of sweet foods and breast cancer risk: a case-control study of women on Long Island, New York. Bradshaw PT, et al. Cancer Causes Control. 2009 Oct;20(8):1509–15.

✦

"A systematic review of published reports identified a total of 37 prospective cohort studies of the glycemic index and glycemic load and chronic disease risk. Significant positive associations were found in validated studies for type 2 diabetes, coronary heart disease, gallbladder disease, and breast cancer."

Glycemic index, glycemic load, and chronic disease risk— a meta-analysis of observational studies. Barclay AW, et al. Am J Clin Nutr. 2008 Mar;87(3):627–37.

✦

"Cases were 2569 women with histologically confirmed incident breast cancer and controls were 2588 women. Information on diet was based on an interviewer-administered questionnaire tested for reproducibility and validity. We found a direct association between breast cancer risk and consumption of sweet foods (including sugar, honey, jam, marmalade, chocolate, cakes, ice cream) with high glycemic index and load, which increase insulin and insulin growth factors."

Consumption of sweet foods and breast cancer risk in Italy. Tavani A. Et al. Ann Oncol. 2006 Feb;17(2):341–5.

✦

"In this population of women ages 20 to 75 years, a high percentage of calories from carbohydrates, but not from fat, was associated with increased breast cancer risk."

Carbohydrates and the risk of breast cancer among Mexican women. Romieu I, et al. Cancer Epidemiol Biomarkers Prev. 2004 Aug;13(8):1283–9.

✦

"In this study among women 20–44 years of age, 568 cases with breast cancer and 1,451 population-based controls were included. Increased risk was observed for high intake of a food group composed of sweet items, particularly sodas and desserts. Risks increased linearly with percent of calories from sweets and frequency of sweets intake."

Increased risk of early-stage breast cancer related to consumption of sweet foods among women less than age 45 in the United States. Potischman N. Coates RJ, et al. Cancer Causes Control. 2002 Dec;13(10):937–46.

✦

"This study support the hypothesis of moderate, direction associations between glycemic index or glycemic load and breast cancer risk, and consequently a possible role of hyperinsulinemia/insulin resistance in breast cancer development."

Dietary glycemic index and glycemic load, and breast cancer *risk: a case-control study.* Augustin LS, et al. Ann Oncol. 2001 Nov;12(11):1533–8.

✦

Significant Colon Cancer Studies:

"This research team, for the first time, looked at whether heavy added sugar consumption might make a difference in colon cancer recurrence. The researchers kept track of over 1000 patients after they had received surgery for colon cancer, taking careful measurements of what they ate and drank. It was found that colon cancer survivors who drank two or more sugar-sweetened beverages per day had an elevated risk of having their colon cancer come back."

Sugar-Sweetened Beverage Intake and Cancer Recurrence. Fuchs MA. Et al. PLOS One. 2014 June 17;9(6): e99816.

✦

"Higher dietary glycemic load and carbohydrate intake were statistically significant associated with an increase risk of recurrence and mortality in stage III colon cancer patients. Our prospective, observational study of 1011 stage III colon cancer patients reported their dietary intake during 6 months."

Dietary glycemic load and cancer recurrence and survival in patients with stage III colon cancer: findings from CALGB

89803. Meyerhardt JA. Et al. J Natl Cancer Inst. 2012 Nov 21;104(22):1702–11.

✦

"Two prospective cohort studies, the Nurses' Health Study and the Health Professional Follow-Up Study, contributed up to 20 years of follow-up; 1,809 incident colorectal cancers were available for analysis. High intakes of glycemic load, fructose, and sucrose were related to an elevated colorectal cancer risk among men. For women, however, these factors did not seem to increase the risk of colorectal cancer."

Dietary glycemic load, carbohydrate, sugar, and colorectal cancer risk in men and women. Michaud DS, et al. Cancer Epidemiol Biomarkers Prev. 2005 Jan;14(1):138–47.

✦

"High consumption of vegetables and fruits and the avoidance of highly refined sugar containing foods are likely to reduce the risk of colon cancer."

Dietary factors and risk of colon cancer. Giovannucci E, Willett WC. Ann Med. 1994 Dec;26(6):443–52.

✦

"A case-control study on colorectal cancer conducted in Italy; cases included 1,125 men and 828 women with histologically confirmed incident cancer of the colon or rectum. Controls were 2,073 men and 2,081 women hospitalized for acute conditions. The positive associations of glycemic index and load with colorectal cancer suggest a detrimental role of refined carbohydrates in the etiology of the disease."

Dietary glycemic load and colorectal cancer risk.
Franceschi S, et al. Ann Oncol. 2001 Feb;12(2):173–8.

✦

"We have investigated the relation between dietary habits and risk of adenocarcinoma of the small intestine using data from 2 hospital-based case-control studies on intestinal cancers conducted in 6 Italian centres. The risk appeared to be directly related to intake of bread, pasta or rice, sugar, and red meat."

Risk factors for adenocarcinoma of the small intestine.
Negri E. Bosetti C, et al. Int J Cancer. 1999 Jul 19;82(2):171–4.

✦

"Glucose intake was associated with a small and non-significant increase in risk for colorectal cancer. An interaction between sucrose and protein intake was found and the odds ratio for high intakes of sucrose and protein was 6.07."

Sucrose as a risk factor for cancer of the colon and rectum: a case-control study in Uruguay. De Stefani E, et al. Int J Cancer. 1998 Jan 5;75(1):40–4.

✦

"Using data from a population-based case-control study of 1993 cases and 2410 controls we examined the associations between dietary sugars, foods containing high level of sugars, and colon cancer. These findings support previous reports that dietary sugars increase risk of colon cancer, possibly through their impact on plasma glucose levels."

Dietary sugar and colon cancer. Slattery ML. Et al.
Cancer Epidemiol Biomarkers Prev. 1997 Sept;6(9):677–85.

✦

"Data were analyzed from a prospective cohort study of 35,215 Iowa women, aged 55–69 years and without a history of cancer, who completed mailed dietary and other questionnaires. These data support hypotheses that sucrose intake or being tall or obese increases colon cancer risk."

Sugar, meat, and fat intake, and non-dietary risk factors for colon cancer *incidence in Iowa women (United States).* Bostick RM, et al. Cancer Causes Control. 1994 Jan;5(1):38–52.

✦

"The association of refined sugars and colorectal cancers and polyps in three recent case-control studies led us to investigate the effects of sucrose, fructose and glucose on colonic epithelial proliferation and sensitivity to carcinogenesis in mice. We conclude that dietary sucrose and fructose may represent risk factors for colorectal cancer through a direct effect of the sugars on colonic epithelial proliferation."

Sucrose enhancement of the early steps of colon carcinogenesis in mice. Stamp D. Et al. Carcinogensis. 1993 Apr;14(4):777–9.

✦

Significant Endometrial Cancer Studies:

"Consumption of foods high in sugar promotes insulin production, which has been linked to endometrial carcinogenesis. We evaluated the impact of dietary intake of sugary foods and beverages, as well as added sugar and total sugar on endometrial cancer risk in a population-based case-control study, including 424 cases and 398 controls. Women in the highest quartile of added sugar intake had significantly increased endometrial cancer risk. The association with added sugar also became stronger when analyses were restricted to {those who were never} users of hormone replacement therapy."

Consumption of sugary foods and drinks and risk of endometrial cancer. King MG. et al. Cancer Causes Control. 2013 Jul;24(7):1427–36.

✦

"Consumption of high-sugar foods stimulates insulin production, which has been associated with endometrial cancer. We used data from the Swedish Mammography Cohort, including 61,226 women aged 40 to 74 years. During 18.4 years of follow-up, 729 participants were diagnosed with incident endometrial cancer. Total sucrose intake and consumption of sweet buns and cookies was associated with increased risk of endometrial cancer."

Sucrose, high-sugar foods, and risk of endometrial cancer— a population-based cohort study. Friberg E. Et al.
Cancer Epidemiol Biomarkers Prev. 2011 Sep;20(9):1831–7.

✦

"Thirty-nine studies were included in the meta-analysis. This comprehensive meta-analysis of glycemic index and glycemic load and cancer risk suggested an overall direct association with colorectal and endometrial cancer."

Glycemic index, glycemic load, and cancer risk: a meta-analysis.
Gnagnarella P, et al. Am J Clin Nutr. 2008 Jun;87(6):1793–801.

✦

Significant Pancreatic Cancer Studies:

"Sugar-sweetened carbonated beverages (called soft drinks) and juices, which have a high glycemic load relative to other foods and beverages, have been hypothesized as pancreatic cancer risk factors. A prospective cohort analysis was done to examine the association in 60,524 participants of the Singapore Chinese Health Study with up to 14 years of follow-up. Individuals consuming > or =2 soft drinks/wk experienced a statistically significant increased risk of pancreatic cancer compared with individuals who did not consume soft drinks."

Soft drink and juice consumption and risk of pancreatic cancer: the Singapore Chinese Health Study. Mueller NT, et al. Cancer Epidemiol Biomarkers Prev. 2010 Feb;19(2):447–55.

✦

"We examined the association between dietary GI and GL and pancreatic cancer by conducting a hospital-based case-control study in Italy of 326 cases of pancreatic cancer and 652 control patients. Dietary data were obtained with the use of a validated food-frequency questionnaire. GI was positively associated with pancreatic cancer. No significant association was observed between GL and pancreatic cancer. Consumption of sugar, candy, honey and jam was positively associated with pancreatic cancer, whereas consumption of fruit was inversely associated."

Dietary glycemic index and glycemic load and risk of pancreatic cancer: a case-control study. Rossi M, et al. Ann Epidemiol. 2010 Jun;20(6):460–5.

✦

"Our findings show that cancer cells can readily metabolize fructose to increase proliferation. Efforts to reduce refined fructose intake or inhibit fructose-mediated actions may disrupt cancer growth."

Fructose induces transketolase flux to promote pancreatic cancer growth. Liu H. Et al. Cancer Res. 2010 Aug 1;70(15):6368–76.

✦

"Participants in the NIH-AARP Diet and Health Study with high free fructose and glucose intake were at a greater risk of developing pancreatic cancer."

Glycemic index, carbohydrates, glycemic load, and the risk of pancreatic cancer in a prospective cohort study. Jiao L, et al. Cancer Epidemiol Biomarkers Prev. 2009 Apr;18(4):1144–51.

✦

"We conducted a population-based case-control study of 532 cases and 1,701 controls. Among men, greater intakes of total and specific sweets were associated with pancreatic cancer risk. Sweets were not consistently associated with risk among women. Low-calorie soft drinks were associated with increased risk among men only. Of the three sugars assessed (lactose, fructose and sucrose) only the milk sugar lactose was associated with pancreatic cancer risk."

Sweets, sweetened beverages, and risk of pancreatic cancer in a large population-based case-control study. Chan JM, et al. Cancer Causes Control. 2009 Aug;20(6):835–46.

✦

"A food-frequency questionnaire was completed by 77,797 women and men aged 45-83 years who had no previous diagnosis of cancer. The participants were followed from 1997 through June 2005. The consumption of added sugar, soft drinks and sweetened fruit soups or stewed fruit was positively associated with the risk of pancreatic cancer."

Consumption of sugar and sugar-sweetened foods and the risk of pancreatic cancer in a prospective study. Larsson SC. Et al. Am J Clin Nutr. 2006 Nov;84(5):1171–6.

✦

"Our data support other findings that impaired glucose metabolism may play a role in pancreatic cancer etiology. A diet high in glycemic load may increase the risk of pancreatic cancer in women who already have an underlying degree of insulin resistance."

Dietary sugar, glycemic load, and pancreatic cancer risk in a prospective study. Michaud DS. Liu S. Giovannucci E. Willett WC, et al. J Natl Cancer Inst. 2002 Sep 4;94(17):1293–300.

✦

"A total of 179 cases and 239 controls were interviewed. Data on food habits, methods of food preparation and preservation, and related information was obtained through a questionnaire. The study found an increased risk of pancreatic cancer associated with a high consumption of salt, smoked meat, dehydrated food, fried food, and refined sugar. An inverse association was found with the consumption of food with no preservatives or additives, raw food, and food prepared by presto or high-pressure cooking."

Food habits and pancreatic cancer: a case-control study of the Francophone community in Montreal, Canada. Ghadirian P, et al. Cancer Epidemiol Biomarkers Prev. 1995 Dec;4(8):895–9.

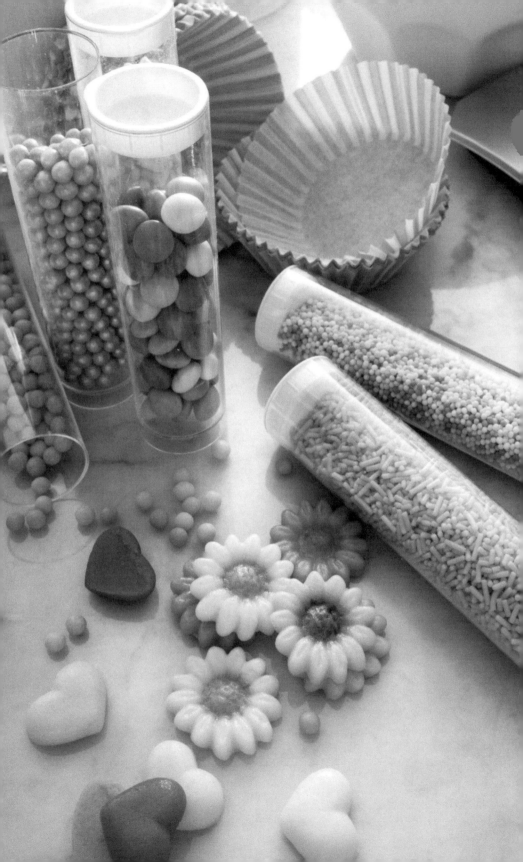

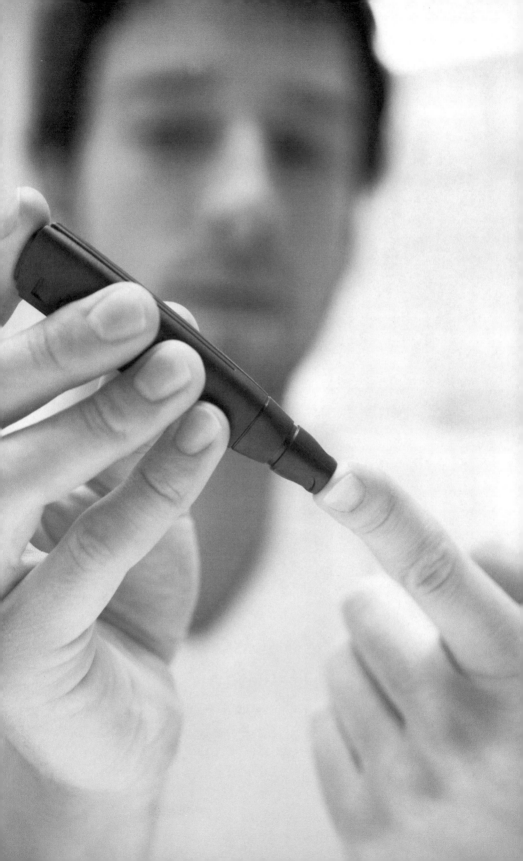

Chapter Four

Diabetes Has
a Sugar Connection

For decades, traditional mainstream medical science has been obsessed with the idea that obesity is the main factor, if not the only important factor, for the onset of diabetes. The more weight a person gains, went this reasoning, the higher that person's risk for developing type 2 diabetes.

There isn't any doubt that being overweight ends up subjecting the human body to multiple health repercussions. But it wasn't until February 2013 that a medical journal, PLoS One, evaluated the study literature covering 175 countries and reached a more important conclusion about the role of body fat and sugars in causing diabetes: Sugar can cause diabetes, irrespective of obesity. In other words, obesity doesn't always lead to diabetes, and sugar intake is a more predictive factor.

No study can ever be "more conclusive than this one," one of the co-authors told *The New York Times*. Every factor imaginable was taken into consideration: poverty, aging, obesity, physical activity levels, total calories consumed, foods eaten, etc. The findings were clearcut—the more sugar available in a nation's diet, the higher the occurrence of diabetes. Your body treats sugar calories differently from fat calories and this makes the various forms of sugar the primary trigger for diabetes.[57]

To give you an example of how this works statistically, these study authors found in their worldwide exhaustive review of the medical literature that for every 12 ounce sugar-sweetened beverage consumed per day per person, the rate of diabetes in that country goes up ONE PERCENT.

This statistic held true whether the people in each country consumed more high-fructose corn syrup or more cane sugar. Table sugar and high-fructose corn syrup activated the same diabetes pathways with equal force.[58]

Subsequent studies teased out even more details. For example, a Mayo Clinic study in 2015 found that added fructose in human diets, as a constituent of added sucrose or as the main component of high-fructose sweeteners, drove up diabetes and diabetes-related metabolic abnormalities over the past decade. "There is no need for added fructose or any added sugars in the diet," warned the study authors.[59]

Both Sugar-Sweetened and Artificially-Sweetened Drinks Guilty

By far the largest source of added sugars (which includes both table sugar and high-fructose corn syrup) in the North American diet comes from sugar-sweetened beverages—soft drinks, sports drinks, energy drinks, and tea and coffee to which sweeteners have been added.

Statistics paint a large part of this disturbing health story.

According to the Centers for Disease Control, from 1980 to 2011 the diagnosed cases of diabetes in the U.S. increased 167% for people below 44 years of age, though almost comparable increases were recorded for all age groups.

During that same period, obesity prevalence increased nearly three-fold until by 2010, 35.5% of U.S. adults were classified as obese.

It is certainly no coincidence that during the same time frame that diabetes and obesity became a documented contagion, consumption of sugar-sweetened beverages increased 135% among all age groups.[60]

Consider how closely the statistics track each other: a 167% diabetes increase during the same general time period as a 135% increase in sugar-sweetened beverage intake.

Studies reported over the past decade further sealed the direct connection between sugar consumption and diabetes risk. This was true worldwide.

European researchers studying hundreds of adolescents in 2013 found that markers for diabetes, such as insulin resistance, became measurably elevated in those who consumed sugar-sweetened beverages five times a week versus those who drank them two or so times a week. The frequency of consumption was directly linked to an increased risk for diabetes.[61]

Published in the *British Journal of Nutrition*, a team of scientists examined medical studies from dozens of countries in 2014 and compared the results, finding an unmistakable pattern of both sugar-sweetened and artificially-sweetened beverages sharply raising type 2 diabetes risks.[62]

More intensive analysis of the study literature in the journal *Obesity Review* turned up more specifics about the risks: just one to two servings a day of sugar-sweetened beverages raises the overall type 2 diabetes risk by 26% compared to drinking just one such beverage a week.[63]

Hidden Sugars in Alcoholic Drinks Are Often Overlooked

Some of the self-professed 'healthiest' eaters, people who are vegetarians or vegans and believe they are effectively managing their sugar intake, make a serious mistake by drinking alcohol in any form and thinking this is not having an impact on their risk for developing diabetes and other health problems.

Most people have absolutely no idea how much sugar lurks inside those alcoholic drinks. And despite what some of you may choose to believe, it's not just beer that provides the highest sugar content and calories to inflate your waistline.

A March 2014 report released by the World Health Organization advised adults to consume no more than 25 grams of sugar a day from all sources, about six teaspoons. Many people absorb more than that in the alcohol they consume on a daily basis as a so-called 'social' drinker.

- Apple cider (alcoholic): 20.5 grams of sugar in a pint. (0.72 ounce)

- Port wine: 20 grams of sugar per glass. (0.70 ounce)

- Bailey's Irish Cream: 19.5 grams per 100 ml. (0.68 ounce)

- Sherry: 9.5 grams per 100 ml. (0.33 ounce)

- Gordon Gin: 14 grams per 250 ml. (0.49 ounce)

- Ale beers: 5 grams per 500 ml. bottle. (0.17 ounce)

- Merlot wine: 2 grams per glass. (0.07 ounce)

- Champagne: 1.5 grams per glass. (0.05 ounce)

The human body treats the presence of alcohol as if it were a nasty chemical toxin; that helps to explain why inebriation produces headaches, fatigue and other symptoms in the body after this alcohol has been absorbed.[64]

After drinking an alcoholic beverage, your blood sugar levels drop. This can be particularly dangerous if you exercise before drinking alcohol because exercise also lowers blood sugar levels. What this effect does is to produce cravings for sugary and carbohydrate-laden foods, making alcohol a trigger for repeated cycles of overeating and addictive sugar consumption.[65]

Finally, I want to share with you the abstract of a report by Dr. Robert Lustig, one of the pioneers in warning about the dangers of sweeteners, who has drawn a link between fructose and alcohol in their related effects on the body.

Fructose: it's alcohol without the buzz. Lustig RH1. Advances in Nutrition. 2013 Mar 1;4(2):226-35. doi: 10.3945/an.112.002998. "What do the Atkins Diet and the traditional Japanese diet have in common? The Atkins Diet is low in carbohydrate and usually high in fat; the Japanese diet is high in carbohydrate and usually low in fat. Yet both work to promote weight loss. One commonality of both diets is that they both eliminate the monosaccharide fructose. Sucrose (table sugar) and its synthetic sister high fructose corn syrup consist of 2 molecules, glucose and fructose. Glucose is the molecule that when polymerized forms starch, which has a high glycemic index, generates an insulin response, and is not particularly sweet. Fructose is found in fruit{and yet it} does not generate an insulin response, and is very sweet. Fructose consumption has increased worldwide, paralleling the obesity and chronic metabolic disease pandemic. Sugar (i.e., fructose-containing mixtures) has been vilified by nutritionists for ages as a source of "empty calories," no different from any other empty calorie. However, fructose is unlike glucose. In the hypercaloric glycogen-replete state, intermediary metabolites from fructose metabolism overwhelm hepatic mitochondrial capacity, which promotes de novo lipogenesis and leads to hepatic insulin resistance, which drives chronic metabolic disease. Fructose also promotes reactive oxygen species formation, which leads to cellular dysfunction and aging, and promotes changes in the brain's reward system, which drives excessive consumption. Thus, fructose can exert detrimental health effects beyond its calories and in ways that mimic those of ethanol, its metabolic cousin. Indeed, the only distinction is that because fructose is not metabolized in the central nervous system, it does not exert the acute neuronal depression experienced by those imbibing ethanol. These metabolic and hedonic analogies argue that fructose should be thought of as "alcohol without the buzz."

More Evidence for
the Sugars/Diabetes Link

Adult rhesus monkeys were fed a high-sucrose diet and in just six months of feeding developed hyperglycemia, hypersinsulinemia, hyperlipidemia, and obesity.

Type 2 Diabetes Mellitus Non-genetic Rhesus Monkey Model Induced by High Fat and High Sucrose Diet. Lu SY. Et al. Exp Clin Endocrinol Diabetes. 2014 Oct 14 {Epub ahead of print}

✦

"A metabolic profile indicating increased risk of diabetes mellitus and cardiovascular disease was observed in animals given access to sugar-sweetened beverages. Notably 'free' fructose {as in high-fructose corn syrup} disrupted glucose homeostasis more than did 'bound' fructose, thus posing a greater risk of progression to type 2 diabetes."

Metabolic and behavioural effects of sucrose and fructose/ glucose drinks in the rat. Sheludiakova A, et al. Eur J Nutr. 2012 Jun;51(4):445–54.

✦

Sugar-sweetened beverages include the full spectrum of soft drinks, fruit drinks, energy and vitamin water drinks, are composed of sucrose, high fructose corn syrup, or fruit juice concentrates. These "promote weight gain and contribute to increased risk of type 2 diabetes and cardiovascular risk factors."

Sweeteners and Risk of Obesity and Type 2 Diabetes: The Role of Sugar-Sweetened Beverages. Malik VS, Hu FB. Curr Diab Rep. 2012 Jan 31 {Epub ahead of print}

✦

"The authors examined the association between soft drinks and juice and the risk of type 2 diabetes among Chinese Singaporeans enrolled in a prospective cohort study of 43,580 participants aged 45–74 years and free of diabetes and other chronic diseases at baseline. Participants consuming 2 soft drinks per week had a relative risk of type 2 diabetes of 1.42 compared with those who rarely consumed soft drinks. Similarly, consumption of 2 juice beverages per week was associated with an increased risk. Relatively frequent intake of soft drinks and juice is associated with an increased risk for development of type 2 diabetes in Chinese men and women."

Soft drink and juice consumption and risk of physician-diagnosed incident type 2 diabetes: the Singapore Chinese Health Study. Odegaard AO, et al. Am J Epidemiol. 2010 Mar 15;171(6):701–8.

✦

"Sugar-sweetened beverages (SSBs) are beverages that contain added caloric sweeteners such as sucrose, high-fructose corn syrup or fruit-juice concentrates, all of which result in similar metabolic effects. They include the full spectrum of soft drinks, carbonated soft drinks, fruitades, fruit drinks, sports drinks, energy and vitamin water drinks, sweetened iced tea, cordial, squashes and lemonade, which collectively are the largest contributor to added sugar intake in the US. Only recently have large epidemiological studies been able to quantify the relationship between SSB consumption and long-term weight gain, type 2 diabetes and cardiovascular disease risk. Experimental studies have provided important insight into potential underlying biological mechanisms. It is thought that SSBs contribute to weight gain in part by incomplete compensation for energy of subsequent meals following intake of liquid calories. They may also increase risk of type 2 diabetes and cardiovascular disease as a contributor to a high dietary glycemic load leading to inflammation, insulin resistance and impaired beta-cell function. Additional metabolic effects from the fructose fraction of these beverages may also promote accumulation of visceral adiposity, and increased hepatic de novo lipogenesis, and hypertension due to hyperuricemia. Consumption of SSBs should therefore be replaced by healthy alternatives such as water, to reduce risk of obesity and chronic diseases."

Sugar-sweetened beverages and risk of obesity and type 2 diabetes: epidemiologic evidence. Hu FB, Malik VS. Physiol Behav. 2010 Apr 26;100(1):47–54.

✦

"We identified 11 studies for inclusion in a random effects meta-analysis comparing sugar-sweetened beverage intake in the highest to lowest quantiles in relation to risk of metabolic syndrome and type 2 diabetes. Based on data from these studies, including 310,819 participants and 15,043 cases of type 2 diabetes, individuals in the highest quantile of sugar-sweetened beverage intake (most often 1–2 servings/day) had a 26% greater risk of developing type 2 diabetes than those in the lowest quantile. In addition to weight gain, higher consumption of sugar-sweetened beverages is associated with development of metabolic syndrome and type 2 diabetes. These data provide empirical evidence that intake of sugar-sweetened beverages should be limited."

Sugar Sweetened Beverages and Risk of Metabolic Syndrome and Type 2 Diabetes: A Meta-analysis. Malik VS, et al. Diabetes Care. 2010 Aug 6. {Epub ahead of print}.

✦

"Many concerns about the health hazards of calorie-sweetened beverages, including soft drinks and fruit drinks and the fructose they provide, have been voiced over the past 10 years. These concerns are related to higher energy intake, risk of obesity, risk of diabetes, risk of cardiovascular disease, risk of gout in men, and risk of metabolic syndrome. Fructose appears to be responsible for most of the metabolic risks, including high production of lipids, increased thermogenesis, and higher blood pressure associated with sugar or high fructose corn syrup. Some claim that sugar is natural, but natural does not assure safety."

Fructose: pure, white, and deadly? Fructose, by any other name, is a health hazard. Bray GA. J Diabetes Sci Technol. 2010 Jul 1:4(4):1003–7.

✦

"A systematic review of published reports identified a total of 37 prospective cohort studies of glycemic index and glycemic load and chronic disease risk. Significant positive associations were found in validated studies for type 2 diabetes, coronary heart disease, gallbladder disease, and breast cancer."

Glycemic index, glycemic load, and chronic disease risk—a meta-analysis of observational studies. Barclay AW, et al. Am J Clin Nutr. 2008 Mar;87(3):627–37.

✦

"We performed a cross sectional study involving a group of 1,018 men and women sampled in the south of Ireland. Participants completed a detailed health and lifestyle questionnaire and provided fasting blood samples for analysis. A lower intake of meat (red meat), meat products, sweets, high fat dairy and white bread (white bread and unrefined cereal) may be associated with enhanced insulin sensitivity and a lower risk of type 2 diabetes."

Prudent diet and the risk of insulin resistance. Villegas R, et al. Nutr Metab Cardiovasc Dis. 2004 Dec;14(6):334–43.

✦

"Carbohydrates with high glycemic indexes and high glycemic loads produce substantial increases in blood glucose and insulin levels after ingestion. The continued intake of high-glycemic-load meals is associated with an increased risk of chronic diseases such as obesity, cardiovascular disease, and diabetes."

Low-glycemic-load diets: impact on obesity and chronic diseases. Bell SJ, et al. Crit Rev Food Sci Nutr. 2003;43(4):357–77.

✦

"Participants were 42,504 male health professionals, 40 to 75 years of age, without diagnosed diabetes at baseline. Using a food frequency questionnaire analysis, a 'western' diet characterized by higher consumption of red meat, processed meat, French fries, high-fat dairy products, refined grains, and sweets and desserts is associated with a substantially increased risk for type 2 diabetes in men."

Dietary patterns and risk for type 2 diabetes mellitus in U.S. men. Van Dam RM, et al. Ann Intern Med. 2002 Feb 5;136(3):201–9.

CHART THREE: Is Your Pancreas a Sugar Sponge?

Where is the pancreas? Located behind the lower part of your stomach in front of your spine, it's a multi-purpose six-inch long gland that is attached to a portion of your small intestine.

Why is it important? Five hormones are secreted by your pancreas to perform necessary functions in the body: **insulin**, which helps to regulate blood sugar levels by transporting glucose; **gastrin**, which assists in your digestion by stimulating your stomach to produce acid; **glucagon**, which stimulates your cells to release glucose, a process that aids insulin in maintaining blood glucose levels; **somatostatin**, which is released if other hormone levels get too high; **vasoactive intestinal peptide**, a hormone which stimulates intestinal cells to release water and salts to aid in digestion.

What disorders affect your pancreas? Pancreatic cancer is one of the more deadly forms of that disease, though it's not the most common problem to affect this organ. Both types 1 and 2 diabetes are much more common disorders. **Type 1 diabetes** occurs when your body fails to produce insulin to manage glucose; **Type 2 diabetes** is the inability of the body to use insulin properly. Hyperglycemia results from the over-production of glucagon creating higher than normal blood

a hormone that stimulates cells to release GLUCOSE

glucose levels; **Hypoglycema** is a low blood glucose level resulting from overproduction of insulin.

Risk factors for pancreatic disorders: Beyond a genetic risk some people inherit, eating fatty foods and absorbing sugars from all sources puts you at greatest risk of having your pancreas go awry. High-fat and carbohydrate diets seem to have a synergistic effect with high alcohol intake, being overweight, and a sedentary lifestyle seem to produce the worst chronic cases of pancreatic disorder. If you eat too much sugar, it can build up in your bloodstream and more readily enter the cells of your body, especially your liver, with help from insulin.

Preventive and treatment options using diet: Whether it's the Mayo Clinic or any other mainstream medical institution, there is general agreement that if you want to prevent pancreatic disorders or treat them, you need to adopt a diet lowering or eliminating refined carbohydrates, sweets, and fatty foods of all kinds. My strong advice is that your emphasis should be on *elimination* of those triggers.

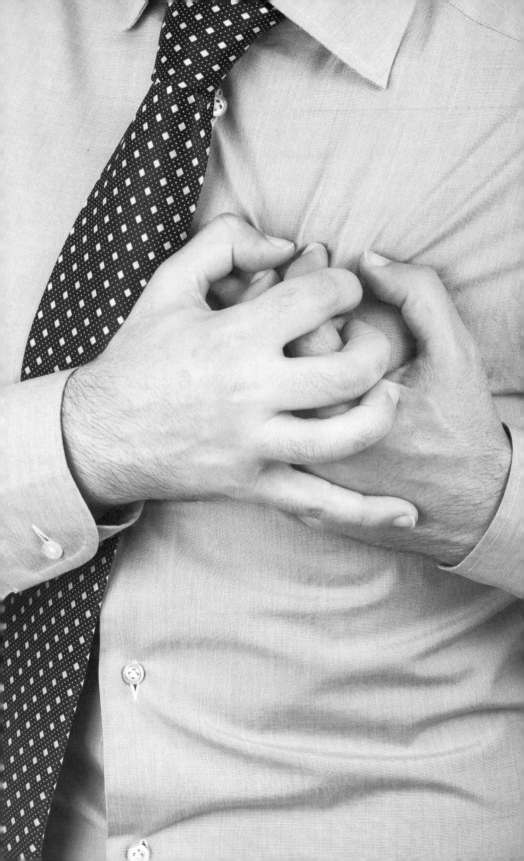

Chapter Five

Heart Attacks, Cardiovascular Disease, Hypertension, Stroke— The Sugar Connection

Y ou can die of heart disease from eating too much sugar.

You didn't know that?

Neither do most cardiologists.

"I spent thirty years working as a cardiologist without ever once wondering what impact sugar had on the heart," declared a cardiologist, Dr. Jeff Ritterman, in 2014. "I wasn't alone in that."[66]

It used to be that most scientists and physicians believed sugar to be bad for your health only because it triggered weight gain which would, in turn, heighten your risk of developing diabetes, heart disease, and a range of other ailments. Many so-called medical experts still believe that, though now the evidence is in that we should know better—eating sugar can kill you directly, not just indirectly through weight gain.

A group of scientists associated with the U.S. Centers for Disease Control and Prevention released a study in 2014 that found the most persuasive link ever between diets high in sugar and the onset of cardiovascular disease. **This finding held up irrespective of whether people were overweight or not.**[67]

These findings came from monitoring more than 31,000 persons between 1988 and 2010 in the National Health and Nutrition Examination Survey. It was by far the most comprehensive look at sugar and the cardiovascular system ever conducted in a medical study.

Anyone who consumes 18 teaspoons or more a day of sugars from all sources significantly elevates their risk for cardiovascular disease, according to the study findings, which estimated that the average American, as well as most Europeans, eats at least 22 teaspoons of sugar per day. Drinking just one name-brand soda injects about nine teaspoons of sugar into the bloodstream.

For the purposes of this study, cardiovascular disease was defined broadly as any chronic disease of the heart, from blood vessel and blood supply problems to the heart, heart valve problems, or an impaired electrical system in the heart muscle.

"Overall, the odds of dying from heart disease rose in tandem with the percentage of sugar in the diet—and that was true regardless of a person's age, sex, physical activity level, and body-mass index," observed the *Harvard Heart Letter*, a publication of Harvard Medical School.[68]

Even if you maintain an otherwise 'healthy' diet of fruits and vegetables and little or no meat and dairy products, should you eat 18 teaspoons or more a day of sugar your risk of dying from cardiovascular disease goes way up.

Sugars are 'empty' calories without fiber, minerals, vitamins or any essential nutrient for a healthy diet. But beyond that, what is the mechanism for how sugar causes cardiovascular disease? Right now the scientific speculation centers on the role that sugar plays in raising blood pressure and causing the liver to rapidly release harmful fats into your bloodstream. Keep in mind that sugar consumption also can trigger fatty liver disease, further accelerating the dumping of harmful fats into the blood. Also keep in mind that fruit sugar is the only type that acts exactly like fat in your system.

More Evidence for the
Sugar & Blood Circulatory System Link

Cardiovascular Disease fruit sugar see p 42

"Fructose, a common nutrient in the westernized diet, has been reported to be associated with increased cardiovascular disease risk. We designed a 4-week randomized, controlled, double-blinded beverage intervention study with 24 overweight Hispanic-American adolescents. Reduction of fructose improves several important factors related to cardiovascular disease."

Dietary fructose reduction improves markers of cardiovascular disease risk in Hispanic-American adolescents with NAFLD. Jin R. Et al. Nutrients. 2014 Aug 8;6(8):31870–201.

✦

"We reviewed the epidemiological, biochemical and psychological evidence that implicates excess sugar intake as an important cause of ill-health. We found relatively consistent evidence of association between markers of sugar intake and risk factors for cardiovascular disease, or the disease itself. We also found some evidence of a sugar addiction syndrome."

Sugar restriction: the evidence for a drug-free intervention to reduce cardiovascular disease risk. Thornley S. Et al. Intern Med J. 2012 Oct;42 Suppl 5:46–58.

✦

The dietary intake of fructose-rich sugar-sweetened beverages has a significant role in raising serum uric acid levels as well as the risk of contracting gout and cardiovascular disease risk factors.

Effects on uric acid, body mass index and blood pressure in adolescents of consuming beverages sweetened with high-fructose corn syrup. Lin WT, et al. Int J Obes. 2012 Aug 14 {Epub ahead of print}

✦

"The consumption of sucrose-sweetened soft drinks has been associated with obesity, the metabolic syndrome, and cardiovascular disorders in observational and short-term intervention studies. We compared the effects of sucrose-sweetened soft drinks with those of isocaloric milk and a noncaloric soft drink on changes in total fat mass and ectopic fat disposition in liver and muscle tissue. Daily intake of sucrose-sweetened soft drinks for 6 months increases ectopic fat accumulation and lipids and is likely to enhance the risk of cardiovascular and metabolic diseases."

Sucrose-sweetened beverages increase fat storage in the liver, muscle, and visceral fat depot: a 6-mo randomized intervention study. Maersk M, et al. Am J Clin Nutr. 2012 Feb;95(2):283–9.

✦

Sugar-sweetened beverages include the full spectrum of soft drinks, fruit drinks, energy and vitamin water drinks, are composed of sucrose, high fructose corn syrup, or fruit juice concentrates. These "promote weight gain and contribute to increased risk of type 2 diabetes and cardiovascular risk factors."

Sweeteners and Risk of Obesity and Type 2 Diabetes:
The Role of Sugar-Sweetened Beverages. Malik VS, Hu FB.
Curr Diab Rep. 2012 Jan 31 {Epub ahead of print}

✦

"A positive association was observed between glucose and diastolic blood pressure with the intake of soft drinks/sweetened beverages, insulin concentrations and the intake of white (processed) bread, and triglyceride concentrations with the intake of added fats."

Correlates of dietary energy sources with cardiovascular disease
risk markers in Mexican school-age children. Perichart-Perera O,
et al. J Am Diet Assoc. 2010 Feb;110(2):253–60.

✦

"Many concerns about the health hazards of calorie-sweetened beverages, including soft drinks and fruit drinks and the fructose they provide, have been voiced over the past 10 years. These concerns are related to higher energy intake, risk of obesity, risk of diabetes, risk of cardiovascular disease, risk of gout in men, and risk of metabolic syndrome. Fructose appears to be responsible for most of the metabolic risks, including high production of lipids, increased thermogenesis, and higher blood pressure associated with sugar or high fructose corn syrup. Some claim that sugar is natural, but natural does not assure safety."

Fructose: pure, white, and deadly? Fructose, by any other name, is a health hazard. Bray GA. J Diabetes Sci Technol. 2010 Jul 1:4(4):1003–7.

✦

"Soft drink consumption is now considered to be a major public health concern with implications for cardiovascular diseases. This follows a number of studies performed in animals suggesting that chronic consumption of refined sugars can contribute to metabolic and cardiovascular dysregulation. In particular, the monosaccharide fructose has been attracting increasing attention as the more harmful sugar component in terms of weight gain and metabolic disturbances. High-fructose corn syrup is gradually replacing sucrose as the main sweetener in soft drinks and has been blamed as a potential contributor to the current high prevalence of obesity. There is also considerable evidence that fructose, rather than glucose, is the more damaging sugar component in terms of cardiovascular risk."

Sugary drinks in the pathogenesis of obesity and cardiovascular diseases. Brown CM, et al. Int J Obes (Lond). 2008 Dec;32 Suppl 6:S28–34.

✦

"Endothelial dysfunction is one of the mechanisms
linking diet and the risk of cardiovascular disease.
Markers of inflammation and endothelial dysfunction
include C-reactive protein, interleukin 6, E-selectin,
sVCAM and SICAM. We conducted a cross-sectional
study of 732 women from the Nurses' Health
Study I cohort who were 43–69 y of age and free of
cardiovascular disease, cancer, and diabetes mellitus.
Dietary intake was documented by using a validated
food-frequency questionnaire in 1986 and 1990. A
Western pattern diet characterized by higher intakes
of red and processed meats, sweets, desserts, French
fries, and refined grains showed a positive relation with
CRP, interleukin, E-selectin, sICAM and sVCAM.
This study suggests a mechanism for the role of dietary
patterns in the pathogenesis of cardiovascular disease."

*Major dietary patterns are related to plasma concentrations of
markers of inflammation and endothelial dysfunction.* Lopez-Garcia
E, et al. Am J Clin Nutr. 2004 Oct;80(4):1029–35.

✦

"Carbohydrates with high glycemic indexes and high
glycemic loads produce substantial increases in blood
glucose and insulin levels after ingestion. The continued
intake of high-glycemic-load meals is associated with

an increased risk of chronic diseases such as obesity, cardiovascular disease, and diabetes."

Low-glycemic-load diets: impact on obesity and chronic diseases. Bell SJ, Sears B. Crit Rev Food Sci Nutr. 2003;43(4):357–77.

✦

"This was a prospective cohort of 44,875 men aged 40-75 y without diagnosed cardiovascular disease or cancer at baseline. During 8 y of follow-up, we documented 1,089 cases of CHD. The Western dietary pattern characterized by higher intake of red meat, processed meat, refined grains, sweets and dessert, French fries and high-fat dairy products predict the risk of coronary heart disease independent of other lifestyle variables."

Prospective study of major dietary patterns and risk of coronary heart disease in men. Hu FB, et al. Am J Clin Nutr. 2000 Oct;72(4):912–21.

Coronary Heart disease

We used data from a prospective 20-y cohort of 2,774 adults. Beverage intake was assessed across years 0 and 7. Higher sugar sweetened beverage consumption was associated with higher risk of high waist circumference, high LDL cholesterol, high triglycerides, and hypertension. Our findings suggest that higher

sugar sweetened beverage consumption is associated
with cariometabolic risk."

*Drinking caloric beverages increases the risk of adverse
cardiometabolic outcomes in the Coronary Artery Risk Development
in Young Adults (CARDIA) Study.* Duffey KJ. Gordon-Larsen P,
et al. Am J Clin Nutr. 2010 Aug 11 {Epub ahead of print}.

✦

"A systematic review of published reports identified
a total of 37 prospective cohort studies of glycemic
index and glycemic load and chronic disease risk.
Significant positive associations were found in validated
studies for type 2 diabetes, coronary heart disease,
gallbladder disease, and breast cancer."

*Glycemic index, glycemic load, and chronic disease risk—
a meta-analysis of observational studies.* Barclay AW, et al.
Am J Clin Nutr. 2008 Mar;87(3):627–37.

Heart attacks

"Male Wistar rats, 21 days old at the start, were
observed for 8 weeks while consuming fructose.
Metabolic and cardiovascular parameters were
measured. Data suggest that early exposure to high
fructose intake produced marked alterations in metabolic
and cardiovascular function, with cardiac damage."

*Early developmental exposure to high fructose intake in rats
causes cardiac damage.* Araujo IC. Et al. Eur J Nutr. 2015 Jan 7.
{Epub ahead of print.}

Hypertension

"Overconsumption of sugar-sweetened beverages has been implicated in the pathogenesis of cardiovascular disease. The objective of the present study was to elucidate acute haemodynamic and microcirculatory responses to the ingestion of sugary drinks. Ingestion of fructose was found to increase blood pressure in healthy human subjects."

Cardiovascular responses to the ingestion of sugary drinks using a randomized cross-over study design: Does glucose attenuate the blood pressure-elevating effect of fructose? Grasser EK. Et al. Br J Nutr. 2014 Jul;112(2):183–92.

✦

"Processed foods happen to be generally high in added sugars, the consumption of which might be strongly and directly associated with hypertension and cardiometabolic risk. Evidence from epidemiological studies and experimental trials in animals and humans suggests that added sugars, particularly fructose, may increase blood pressure and blood pressure variability."

The wrong white crystals: not salt but sugar as aetiological in hypertension and cardiometabolic disease. DNicontantonio JJ. Et al. Open Heart. 2014;1:doi:10,1136.

✦

"We used data from a prospective 20-y cohort of 2,774 adults. Beverage intake was assessed across years 0 and 7. Higher sugar sweetened beverage consumption was associated with higher risk of high waist circumference, high LDL cholesterol, high triglycerides, and hypertension. Our findings suggest that higher sugar sweetened beverage consumption is associated with cariometabolic risk."

Drinking caloric beverages increases the risk of adverse cardiometabolic outcomes in the Coronary Artery Risk Development in Young Adults (CARDIA) Study. Duffey KJ, et al. Am J Clin Nutr. 2010 Aug 11 {Epub ahead of print}.

✦

"Reduced consumption of sugar-sweetened beverages and sugars was significantly associated with reduced blood pressure. Such reductions may be an important dietary strategy to lower blood pressure."

Reducing consumption of sugar-sweetened beverages is associated with reduced blood pressure: a prospective study among United States adults. Chen L, et al. Circulation. 2010 Jun 8;121(22):2398–406.

✦

"Overweight subjects who consumed fairly large amounts of sucrose (28% of energy), mostly as beverages, had increased energy intake, body weight, fat mass, and blood pressure after 10 wk. These effects were not observed in a similar group of subjects who consumed artificial sweeteners."

Sucrose compared with artificial sweeteners: different effects on ad libitum food intake and body weight after 10 wk of supplementation in overweight subjects. Raben A, et al. Am J Clin Nutr. 2002 Oct;76(4):721–9.

Sucrose = white table sugar

+

"All substrains showed the highest systolic blood pressure when ingesting the two diets highest in sucrose. High dietary sucrose can chronically increase systolic blood pressure in three substrains of Wistar rats."

Sugar-induced blood pressure elevations over the lifespan of three substrains of Wistar rats. Preuss HG. Zein M, et al. J Am Coll Nutr. 1998 Feb;17(1):36–47.

Stroke

"This study sought to determine the effect of various sugar substitutes on the cerebral ischemic injury and endothelial progenitor cells in mice. Long-term consumption of sugar substitutes aggravated cerebral ischemic injury."

Dietary intake of sugar substitutes aggravates cerebral ischemic injury and impairs endothelial progenitor cells in mice. Dong XH. Et al. Stroke. 2015 Jun;46(6):1714–8.

+

"The nurses' Health Study, a prospective cohort study of 84,085 women followed for 28 years and the Health Professionals Follow-up Study, a prospective cohort study of 43,371 men followed for 22 years, provided data on soda consumption and incident stroke. Greater consumption of sugar-sweetened and low-calorie sodas was associated with a significantly higher risk of stroke."

Soda consumption and the risk of stroke in men and women. Bernstein AM, et al. Am J Clin Nutr. 2012 May;95(5):1190–9.

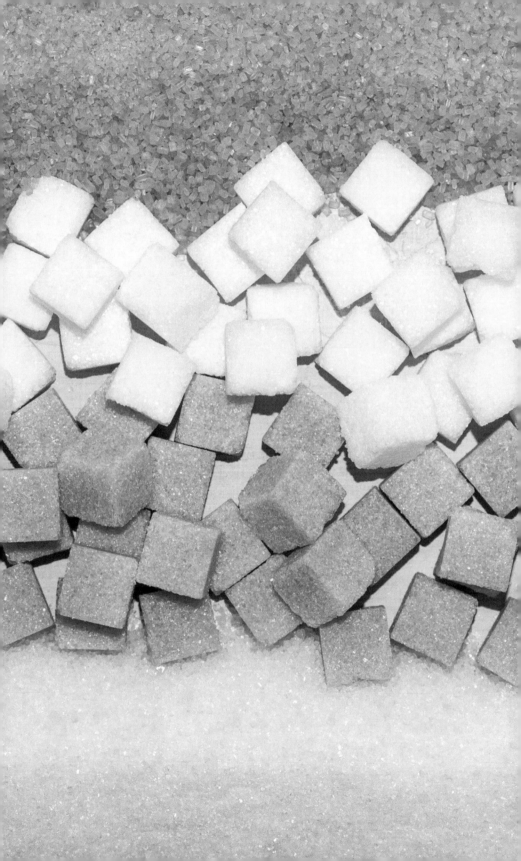

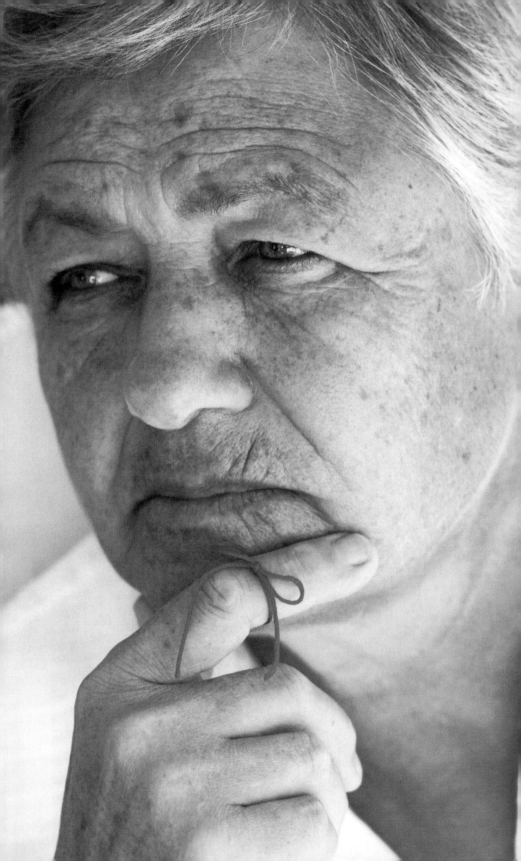

Chapter Six

Your Brain on Sugar Equals Alzheimer's, Depression, Cognitive, Memory and Behavioral Problems

D id you ever wonder why children's documented behavioral problems and learning difficulties became such an epidemic over the past few decades? Look no further than the sweeteners added to their diets, at home and at school, over that same period of time.

Ever wonder why Alzheimer's disease and dementia in general became an epidemic beginning in the 1970s? Look no further than the trend in elevated consumption levels of added sugars over that time period.

How about chronic depression? Did it occur to you that 'sugar on the brain' could be a responsible factor in the onset of depression and a range of other psychiatric disorders, including schizophrenia? If not, think again!

Medical science has learned a lot about sweeteners and the human brain in just the past few years. After neglecting the connection for so long, researchers suddenly began to wake up and see with growing distress what many of us had been warning about. In my case, 1980 marked the year that I, as Director of the Hippocrates Institute, removed all sugar, including fruit, from the diet of those people facing mental or physical challenges.

"It is alarming that commonly consumed low-cost foods with high sugar and fat contents have the potential to determine mental health," commented the authors of a May 2012 scientific report in *The Journal of Physiology*, which examined the impact of added sugars, including high fructose corn syrup, on human brain function.

Most disturbing is the research showing high sucrose diets can have effects on brain function transferred from mother to child in the womb. A 2014 study published in the *Journal of Nutrition & Biochemistry*, for instance, found learning deficits and cognition disorders in offspring born to mothers fed a diet high in sugars. Though this experiment was done with lab animals, the researchers were able to extrapolate the findings to humans with the observation it would explain many of the observed "cognition disorders in young children."[69]

In the *British Journal of Nutrition,* a team of researchers described in 2013 how they studied 40 children, aged 10 to 12 years, after they had consumed glucose beverages. Their cognitive performance, including memory and attention, was monitored each hour. Girls in particular demonstrated memory deficits, recalling fewer words on memory tests than when they just drank water.[70]

Despite the floodgates of research beginning to open on the links between sweeteners and disordered behavior, U.S. government health agencies and those of other countries remain largely behind the curve in accepting or acknowledging these links.

The normally very conservative U.S. National Library of Medicine, a part of the National Institutes of Health, did concede some of the link between added sugars and children's behavior (hyperactivity) in a 2013 post on its website: "Refined (processed) sugars may have some effect on children's activity. Refined sugars and carbohydrates enter the bloodstream quickly. Therefore, they cause rapid changes in blood sugar levels. This may make a child become more active."[71]

Much of the best research on sugar and brain function has occurred outside the U.S., largely beyond the reach of influence by the U.S. food corporations, sugar production interests, and other financial concerns that try to protect their profits by keeping a lid on damaging research findings.

For example, it was a research team in Denmark, at the University of Copenhagen, which found in 2014 a link between refined sugars and mood, not just in children but in adults. Similarly, it was scientists from Serbia, at the University of Belgrade, who published the results of a study showing how high fructose diets produce brain problems, in particular cognitive deficits.

Interestingly, it was a joint French/American team of researchers in 2013 that made a finding about how the spice cinnamon could be used to counteract the memory impairment and other Alzheimer-associated brain changes coming from consumption of high fructose foods and beverages.[72]

Evidence: Alzheimer's Disease & the Role of Sugars

"Preventing or postponing the onset of Alzheimer's disease and delaying or slowing its progression would lead to a consequent improvement of health status and quality of life in older age. Poorer cognitive function and an increased risk of vascular dementia were found to be associated with consumption of milk or dairy products, and a diet high in added sugars."

Diet and Alzheimer's disease risk factors or prevention: the current evidence. Solfrizzi V. Et al. Exp Rev Neurotherapeutics. 2011 May;11(5):677–708.

✦

"Intake of saturated fats and simple carbohydrates (glucose and sucrose), two of the primary components of a modern Western diet, is linked with the development of obesity and Alzheimer's disease. Evidence shows that consumption of a meal containing simple carbohydrates can impair postprandial memory function. It was found that the high glycemic meal led to poorer performance in memory tests given between 1-2 hours after eating."

Western Diet Consumption and Cognitive Impairment: Links to Hippocampal Dysfunction and Obesity. Kanoski SE. Davidson TL. Physiol Behav. 2011 Apr 18;103(1):59–68.

Behavioral problems in children

"Hyperactivity is a very common disorder in children, especially males. Chocolate, sugar, sweeteners, additives, preservatives, dyes, can enhance an incidence of this syndrome."

Attention deficit and infantile hyperactivity. Berdonces JL. Rev Enferm (Spanish). 2001 Jan;24(1):11–4.

✦

"Eating simple sugars has been suggested as having adverse behavioral and cognitive effects in children. This study was performed to address a physiologic mechanism for this effect. Metabolic, hormonal and symptomatic responses to a standard oral glucose load were compared in 25 healthy children and 23 young adults. Enhanced adrenomedullary responses to modest reductions in plasma glucose concentration and increased susceptibility to neuroglycopenia may be important contributing factors to adverse behavioral and cognitive effects after sugar ingestion in healthy children."

Enhanced adrenomedullary response and increased susceptibility to neuroglycopenia: mechanisms underlying the adverse effects of sugar ingestion in healthy children. Jone TW, et al. J Pediatr. 1995 Feb;126(2):171–7.

✦

"The meta-analysis of the studies to date found that sugar does not affect the behavior or cognitive performance of children. The strong belief of parents may be due to expectancy and common association. However, a small effect of sugar or effects on subsets of children cannot be ruled out."

The effect of sugar on behavior or cognition in children. A meta-analysis. Wolraich ML, et al. JAMA. 1995 Nov 22–29;274(20):1617–21.

◆

"On separate mornings each child among eight preschool children received 6 ounces of juice, sweetened on one morning with sucrose and on the other with an artificial sweetener. Following the sucrose drink the children showed a decrement in performance in the structured testing situation and they demonstrated more 'inappropriate' behavior during free play. These differences in behavior were most pronounced approximately 45 to 60 minutes after the drinks."

Behavioral effects of sucrose on preschool children. Goldman JA, et al. J Abnorm Child Psychol. 1986 Dec;14(4):565–77.

Brain Function & Memory Problems

"High fructose diet has been shown to have damaging effects on the hippocampus, a brain region critical for learning and memory. Fructose-induced hippocampal dysfunction may arise from insulin resistance and inflammation. Our results showed that long-term consumption of 10% fructose solution induces hippocampal insulin resistance and inflammation. Rats fed with higher concentrations of fructose displayed impaired plastic responses of the hippocampus which may provide a basis for cognitive deficits."

The impact of different fructose loads on insulin sensitivity, inflammation, and PSA-NCAM-mediated plasticity in the hippocampus of fructose-fed male rats. Djordjevic A. Et al. Nutr Neurosci. 2015 Feb;18(2):66–75.

✦

"The hippocampus plays a crucial role in learning and memory, and neuronal apoptosis in the hippocampus contributes to learning deficits. This study determined the influence of maternal high sucrose diets on behavior and hippocampal neurons in the young offspring. The results demonstrated that prenatal high sucrose diets could induce the spatial acquisition deficits in the young offspring associated with hippocampal apoptosis and might play a critical role in cognition disorders in young children."

Hippocampal apoptosis involved in learning deficits in the offspring exposed to maternal high sucrose diets. Kuang H. Et al. J Nutr Biochem. 2014 Sep;25(9):985–90.

✦

"Here we examined the effects of sucrose and high fructose corn syrup intake during adolescence or adulthood on cognitive and metabolic outcomes. Adolescent or adult male rats were given 30-day access to chow containing either water, sucrose solution, or HFCS (high fructose corn syrup) solution. These data show that consumption of added sugars, particularly

HFCS, negatively impacts hippocampal function, metabolic outcomes, and neuroinflammation."

Effects of sucrose and high fructose corn syrup consumption on spatial memory function and hippocampal neuroinflammation in adolescent rats. Hsu TM. Et al. Hippocampus. 2014 Sep 20. {Epub ahead of print.}

✦

"A total of 40 children (10–12 years) completed a double-blind, randomized, crossover trial, receiving three isoenergetic drinks, including a glucose beverage. For three hours post-consumption, subjective appetite and cognitive performance (speed of processing, memory, attention and perceptual speed) were measured hourly." After consuming the glucose drink girls demonstrated less word recall with short-term memory deficits.

The effect of beverages varying in glycaemic load on postprandial glucose responses, appetite and cognition in 10-12 year old school children. Brindal E. Et al. Br J Nutr. 2013 Aug 28;110(3):529–37.

✦

"Overall dietary energy intake, particularly the consumption of simple sugars such as fructose, has been increasing steadily in Western societies, but the effects on the brain are poorly understood. Here, we used functional and structural assays to characterize the effects of excessive caloric intake on

the hippocampus, a brain region important for learning
and memory. Rats fed with a high-fat, high-glucose diet
supplemented with high-fructose corn syrup showed
alterations in energy and lipid metabolism similar to
clinical diabetes, with elevated fasting glucose and
increased cholesterol and triglycerides. Rats maintained
on this diet for 8 months exhibited impaired spatial
learning ability, reduced hippocampal dendritic spine
density, and reduced long-term potentiation at Schaffer
collateral-CA1 synapses. We conclude that a high-
calorie diet reduces hippocampal synaptic plasticity
and impairs cognitive function."

Diet-induced insulin resistance impairs hippocampal synaptic
plasticity and cognition in middle-aged rats. Stranahan AM, et al.
Hippocampus. 2008;18(11):1085–8.

✦

"We have investigated a potential mechanism by
which a diet, similar in composition to the typical
diet of most industrialized western societies rich in
saturated fat and refined sugar, can influence brain
structure and function via regulation of neurotrophins.
Our results indicate that a popularly consumed diet can
influence crucial aspects of neuronal and behavioral
plasticity associated with the function of brain-derived
neurotrophic factor."

A high-fat, refined sugar diet reduces hippocampal brain-derived neurotrophic factor, neuronal plasticity, and learning. Molteni R, et al. Neuroscience. 2002;112(4):803–14.

Depression

"Major depressive disorder is a debilitating disease in the Western World. A western diet high in saturated fat and refined sugar seems to play an important part in disease development. Our study with 42 mice randomly assigned to one of three experimental diets—a high fat, a high sucrose, or a control diet—for 13 weeks showed that dietary fat and sucrose affect behavior."

A possible link between food and mood: dietary impact on gut microbiota and behavior in BALB/c mice. Pyndt Jorgensen B. Et al. PLoS One. 2014 Aug 18;9(8):e103398.

✦

"Key biological factors that influence the development of depression are modified by diet This study examined the extent to which the high-prevalence mental disorders are related to habitual diet in 1,046 women ages 20-93 years randomly selected from the population. A "western" diet of processed or fried foods, refined grains, sugary products, and beer was associated with higher odds for major depression and anxiety disorders. These results demonstrate an association between habitual diet quality and the high-prevalence mental disorders."

Association of Western and traditional diets with depression and anxiety in women. Jacka FN, et al. Am J Psychiatry. 2010 Mar;167(3):305–11.

Schizophrenia

"A higher national dietary intake of refined sugar and dairy products predicted a worse 2-year outcome of schizophrenia. A high national prevalence of depression was predicted by a lower dietary intake of fish and seafood. The dietary predictors of outcome of schizophrenia and prevalence of depression are similar to those that predict illnesses such as coronary heart disease and diabetes, which are more common in people with mental health problems."

International variations in the outcome of schizophrenia and the prevalence of depression in relation to national dietary practices: an ecological analysis. Peet M. Br J Psychiatry. 2004 May;184:404–8.

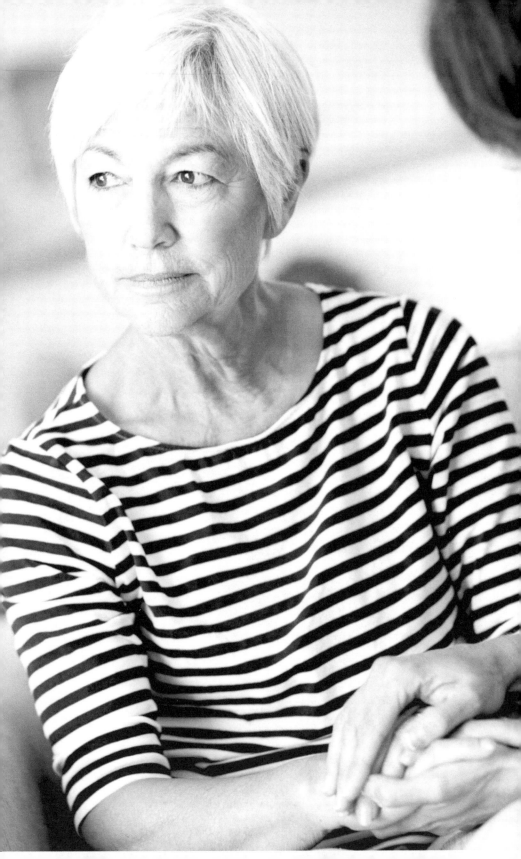

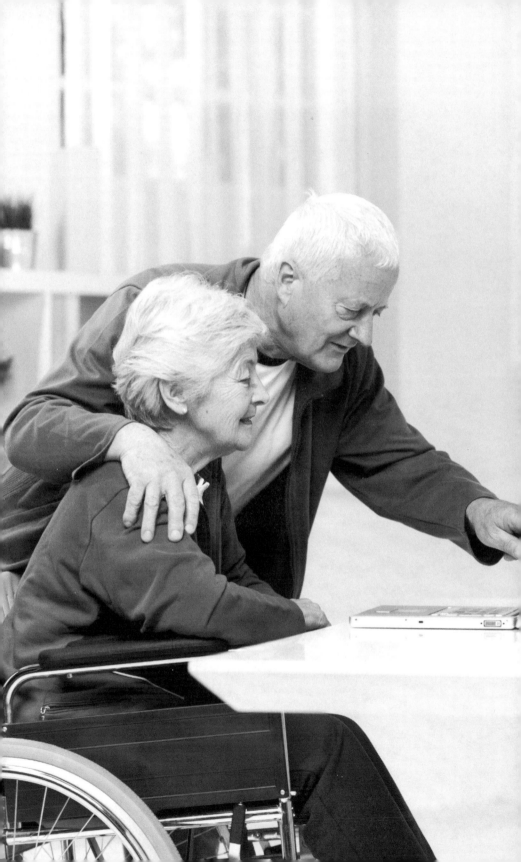

Chapter Seven

Sugars Accelerate Your Aging

An estimated 300 theories of aging have been proposed in the scientific literature and the question of why and how we age continues to be explored and debated with hundreds of new studies each year.

What we do know with some confidence is that sweetener consumption makes you age faster and more visibly, and it can shorten your lifespan.

At first this idea that sugar accelerates aging came in the form of a theory advanced in 2003, in the journal *Medical Hypotheses*. The author evaluated studies done on the benefits of caloric restriction in extending lifespan, and studies done on the health impacts of sugars and fats, to offer a path for future research to investigate whether "restriction of foods with a high glycemic index would avoid or delay many diseases of aging and might result in life extension."[73]

Subsequent research began to establish the links between the various sugars and age acceleration.

Studies detailed how chronic sugar intake produces glycation in the body, which in turn damages collagen and elastin fibers in the skin, which results in sagginess, wrinkles and skin discoloration. The typical signs of aging manifest.

But it gets worse for you sugar eaters. A by-product of glycation are free radicals which not only further contribute to accelerated aging, yet also make the skin more vulnerable to damage from the sun, thus raising the risk of skin cancer. Even greater concentrations of free radicals are generated by consuming high fructose corn syrup.

Sugar intake also shortens your life.

In 2014 a study published in the *American Journal of Public Health* revealed that people who drank sugar-sweetened sodas had shorter telomeres than people who didn't drink them. Telomeres are at the end of chromosomes inside our cells and as these cells divide over time with age, telomeres get shorter, a standard marker for aging. Sugar's impact on telomeres, accelerating this shortening, tells us that sugar promotes faster aging and quicker death.[74]

In another experiment evaluating how other people view the ages of sugar eaters, a team of scientists in Holland in

2013 took photographs of 602 test subjects, men and women aged 50 to 70 years, and measured their non-fasting glucose and insulin levels. These photographs were then shown to a board of 60 independent assessors who were asked to assess the ages of test subjects. The higher the person's blood glucose level, the older that person looked and was rated by the independent viewers.[75]

This was a consistent study finding. Sugar consumption produces high blood glucose levels, which in turn ages the person faster, a phenomenon that is visible to other people.

"We took into account other factors such as whether or not that person smoked and yet still the effects were clear—the higher the blood glucose, the older the person looked," commented Dr. David Gunn, a co-author of the study, in an interview he did with Britain's *The Daily Mail* newspaper.

"Skin experts agree," observed dermatologists quoted in the newspaper article. "A diet high in sugar is a disaster for the face."

An even deadlier combination to accelerate aging and hasten death is to mix a sugar-laden diet with high levels of stress. The stress hormone cortisol was measured in a large group of volunteers in another study by the same Dutch researchers, along with the glucose levels, and another clear trend emerged showing that sugar and cortisol make people older.

It may be a synergistic effect at work between stress and sugar. This is an angle on aging that remains to be fully explored by research scientists, though it already makes perfect sense. We know from a substantial body of research that stress is both a premature age-promoter and a serial killer. Now we know that sugar is, too. Combine the two killers together and we have a criminal gang loose in our lives.

Evidence for the Sugar
and Aging Link

"Glucose and cortisol have been previously associated with facial aging. We assessed a random sample of 579 people from the Leiden Longevity Study. A higher non-fasted glucose level and a higher fasted cortisol level tended to associate with a higher perceived age based on skin wrinkling."

Disentangling the effects of circulating IGF-1, glucose, and cortisol on features of perceived age. Van Drielen K. Et al. Age. 2015 Jun;37(3):9771.

✦

"Wild-derived mice were fed either fructose, glucose or sucrose for 40 weeks. Females fed the fructose and glucose diet experience a mortality rate 1.9 times the rate of controls and produced 26.4% fewer offspring."

Compared to sucrose, previous consumption of fructose and glucose monosaccharides reduces survival and fitness of female mice. Ruff JA. Et a. J Nutr. 2015 Mar;145(3):434–41.

✦

"We tested whether leukocyte telomere length maintenance, which underlies healthy cellular aging, provides a link between sugar-sweetened beverage consumption and the risk of cardiometabolic disease. We examined cross-sectional associations between the consumption of sugar-sweetened beverages, diet soda, and fruit juice and telomere length in a sample of 5309 health US adults aged 20 to 65 years with no history of diabetes or cardiovascular disease. Sugar-sweetened soda consumption was associated with shorter telomeres. Consumption of 100% fruit juice was marginally associated with longer telomeres."

Soda and cell aging: associations between sugar-sweetened beverage consumption and leukocyte telomere length in healthy adults from the National Health and Nutrition Examination Surveys. Leung CW. Et al. Am J Public Health. 2014 Dec;104(12):2425–31.

✦

"Perceived age was assessed using facial photographs and non-fasted glucose and insulin were measured in 602 subjects. In non-diabetic subjects perceived age was increased by 0.40 years per 1 mmol/L increase in glucose level. The present study demonstrates that higher glucose levels are associated with a higher perceived age."

High serum glucose levels are associated with a higher perceived age. Noordam R. Et al.Age. 2013 Feb;35(1):189–95.

✦

"Here we show that comparatively low levels of added sugar consumption have substantial negative effects on mouse survival, competitive ability, and reproduction. We demonstrate that fructose/glucose-fed females experience a twofold increase in mortality."

Human-relevant levels of added sugar consumption increase female mortality and lower male fitness in mice. Ruff JS. Et al. Nat Commun. 2013;4:2245.

✦

"The effect of sugars on aging skin is governed by the simple act of covalently cross-linking two collagen fibers, which renders both of them incapable of easy repair. Glucose and fructose link the amino acids present in the collagen and elastin that support the dermis, producing advanced glycation and products or Ages. This process is accelerated in all body tissues when sugar is elevated and is further stimulated by ultraviolet light in the skin."

Nutrition and aging skin: sugar and glycation.
Danby FW. Clin Dermatol. 2010 Jul–Aug;28(4):409–11.

✦

"Telomeres serve as a mitotic clock and biological marker of senescence. Diabetic mellitus is associated with damage to target organs and premature aging. We assessed the effect of glycemic control on telomere dynamics in arterial cells of 58 patients undergoing coronary artery bypass and in mononuclear blood cells of other diabetic (32 type I) and 47 (type II) patients. Telomeres were significantly shorter in the arteries of diabetic versus non-diabetic patients and in mononuclear cells of both type I and type II diabetes. In all study groups good glycemic control attenuated shortening of the telomeres."

Telomere dynamics in arteries and mononuclear cells of diabetic patients: effectof diabetes and of glycemic control. Uziel O, et al. Exp Gerontol. 2007 Oct;42(10):971–8.

✦

"Sugar-induced negative effects on epidermal keratinocytes, using glucose and glyoxal, with a 3-day treatment, prematurely aged the epidermal keratinocytes."

Sugar-induced premature aging and altered differentiation in human epidermal keratinocytes. Berge U, etal. Ann N Y Acad Sci. 2007 Apr;1100:524–9.

✦

"Telomere shortening is seen even at the stage of impaired glucose tolerance. Among subjects with type 2 diabetes, those with atherosclerotic plaques had greater shortening of telomere length compared to those without plaques."

Association of telomere shortening with impaired glucose tolerance and diabetic macroangiopathy. Adaikalakoteswari A, et al. Atherosclerosis. 2007 Nov;195(1):83–9.

✦

"Our data demonstrated that glucose-induced aging in vitro caused an elongation and thickening of cell processes. A possible age-inducing effect of glucose is also supported by the decrease of ras protein expression and shortening of telomeres."

Exogenous application of glucose induces aging in rat cerebral oligodendrocytes as revealed by alteration in telomere length. Dabouras V. Rothermel A, et al. Neurosci Lett. 2004 Sep 16;368(1):68–72.

✦

"Simultaneous consideration of the influence of the different types of carbohydrates and fats in human diets on mortality rates (especially the diseases of aging) and the probable retardation of such diseases by caloric restriction leads to the hypothesis that restriction of foods with a high glycemic index and saturated or hydrogenated fats would avoid or delay many diseases of aging and might result in life extension."

Does dietary sugar and fat influence longevity? Archer VE. Med Hypotheses. 2003 Jun;60(6):924–9.

✦

"This study addressed whether food and nutrient intakes were correlated with skin wrinkling in a sun-exposed site. 177 Greek-born subjects living in Melbourne, 69 Greek subjects living in rural Greece, 48 Anglo-Celtic Australian elderly living in Melbourne and 159 Swedish subjects living in Sweden, participating in the International Union of Nutritional Science Food Habits in Later Life study, had their dietary intakes measure and their skin assessed. Food and nutrient intakes were assessed using a validated semi-quantitative food frequency questionnaire. Correlation analyses on the pooled data and using the major food groups suggested that there may be less actinic skin damage with a higher intake of vegetables, olive oil, legumes, and lower intake of butter, margarine, milk products, and sugar products."

Skin wrinkling: can food make a difference? Purba MB. Kouris-Blazos A, et al. J Am Coll Nutr. 2001 Feb;20(1):71–80.

✦

"Although critical gaps remain in our understanding of how dietary sucrose can affect biological aging, evidence exists that the type and amounts of dietary carbohydrate can significantly affect the health and life span of elderly people."

Influence of dietary sucrose on biological aging. McDonald RB. Am J Clin Nutr. 1995 Jul;62(1 Suppl):284S–292S.

✦

"Several studies in the last decade have highlighted
the importance of the hexose sugars and especially
glucose, as being responsible for alterations to living
protein and other molecules. The phenomenon of
nonenzymatic glycation—by which the carbonyl group
of glucose can directly condense with a free amino
group—may be relevant to the process of aging and for
the pathogenesis of late diabetic complications."

Advanced nonenzymatic glycation endproducts (AGE):
their relevance to aging and the pathogenesis of late diabetic
complications. Sensi M, et al. Diabetes Res. 1991 Jan;16(1):1–9.

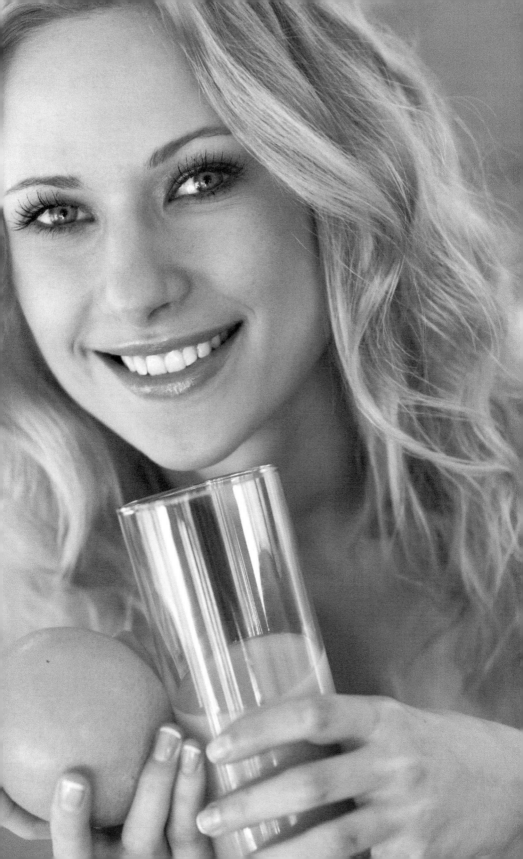

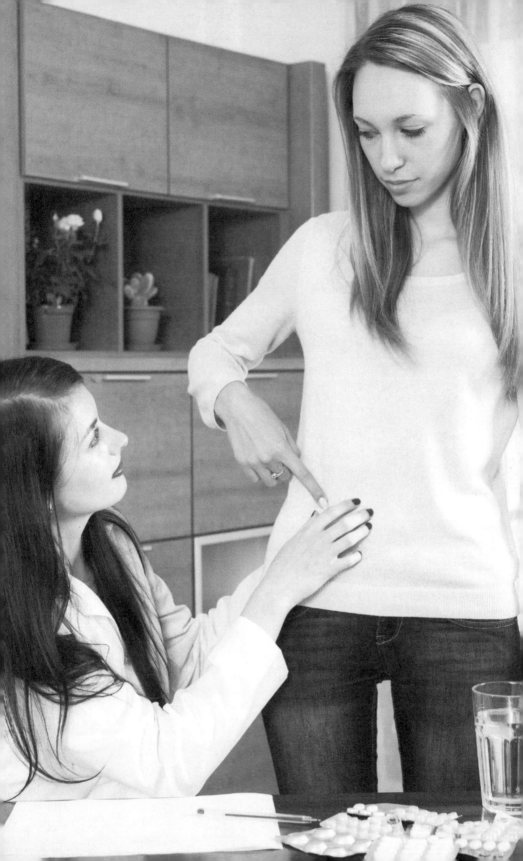

Chapter Eight

Non-Alcoholic Fatty Liver Disease from Sweeteners

I t used to be that fatty liver disease was a serious medical condition primarily seen in alcoholics, but that all began to change over the past three decades as rising fructose consumption triggered a now widespread condition called non-alcoholic fatty liver disease.

This condition occurs when the human liver has difficulty breaking down fats and as a result, these fats accumulate in the liver causing a potentially life-threatening medical situation

for the body. With this liver inflammation comes scarring of
liver tissue and over time, liver failure can develop.

Quite often there are few severe symptoms indicating that
non-alcoholic fatty liver disease (NAFLD) is developing.
Some signs might include recurring pain in the upper right
abdomen and chronic fatigue.

Because fructose is processed in the liver, which isn't the
case with other types of sugars, the liver is overwhelmed by
the amounts of high fructose corn syrup and other types of
fructose now found in Western diets. Small amounts of fructose can be handled by a healthy liver, yet the amounts coming from sweetened beverages and processed foods cannot be
properly processed by even the healthiest of human livers.
Nor can large amounts of fruit or their juices, including fructose rich carrot and beet juice.

Most consumers have no idea how much fructose they are
consuming, much less how dangerous the fructose is to their
health. This ignorance—and the health dangers that accom-
pany it—has been intentionally perpetuated by the processed
food and beverage industries.

A laboratory analysis of 23 popular sweetened beverages
done in 2011 found that manufacturers consistently misled
the public by listing a lower fructose and sugar content on
labels than the products actually contained. Published in the
medical journal *Obesity,* study authors discovered "that the
total sugar content of the beverages ranged up to 128% of
what was listed on the food label."

A direct result of processed foods and beverages being laden with fructose is that 31% of American adults and 13% of children have now developed some degree of non-alcoholic fatty liver disease (NAFLD).[76,77]

Severe cases of NAFLD progress into a condition called non-alcoholic steatohepatitis, in which vital blood flow into the liver is restricted. The non-profit medical science organization SugarScience estimates that up to 6 million people in the U.S. now have this condition (the rates have doubled over just a few decades) and it has become one of the leading reasons for liver transplants.

An added health concern from fructose consumption is development of belly fat, sometimes called 'sugar belly.' As the fat cells accumulate around a person's midsection, hormone imbalances are created in the body. These imbalances hasten the onset of many diseases, ranging from cancer and diabetes to heart disease and even Alzheimer's disease.[78]

More Evidence Linking Sweeteners & Non-Alcoholic Fatty Liver Disease

"We examined the cross-sectional association between intake of sugar-sweetened beverages and fatty liver disease in participants of the Framingham Offspring and Third General cohorts, 5908 participants. We observed that regular sugar-sweetened beverage consumption was associated with greater risk of fatty liver disease, particularly in overweight and obese individuals."

Sugar-sweetened beverage, diet soda, and fatty liver disease in the Framingham Heart Study cohorts. Ma J. Et al. J Hepatol. 2015 May 29;SO168(15)00240–8.

✦

"The objective of this study was to measure fructose absorption/metabolism in pediatric non-alcoholic fatty liver disease (NAFLD) compared with obese and lean controls. Children with histologically proven NAFLD and obese and lean controls received oral fructose. Following fructose ingestion, NAFLD vs. lean controls had elevated serum glucose, insulin and uric acid but lower fructose excretion. Children with NAFLD absorb and metabolize fructose more effectively than lean subjects, associated with an exacerbated metabolic profile following fructose ingestion."

Oral fructose absorption in obese children with non-alcoholic fatty liver disease. Sullivan JS. Et al. Pediatr Obes. 2014 Jun 24 {Epub ahead of print.}

✦

"Fructose intake has increased considerably in recent years, especially in the form of high fructose corn syrup, due to its high sweetening power. This review aims to update the effect of high intake of fructose in the liver and intestine, mainly associated with processed foods with added fructose. Seventy eight articles met the inclusion criteria. Conclusion: high fructose intake has been associated to pathologies as non-alcoholic fatty liver disease and fructose malabsorption."

Fructose consumption and its health implications; fructose malabsorption and nonalcoholic fatty liver disease. Riveros MJ. Et al. Nutr Hosp. 2014 Mar 1;29(3):491–9.

✦

"Growing evidence suggests that fructose contributes to the development and severity of non-alcoholic fatty liver disease. Sufficient evidence exists to support clinical recommendations that fructose intake be limited through decreasing foods and drinks high in add fructose-containing sugars."

Dietary fructose in nonalcoholic fatty liver disease. Vos MB. Lavine JE. Hepatology. 2013 Jun;57(6):2525–31.

✦

"Soft drinks are the leading source of added sugar worldwide and have been linked to obesity, diabetes and metabolic syndrome. The consumption of soft drinks can increase the prevalence of nonalcoholic fatty liver disease. During regular soft drinks consumption, fat accumulates in the liver by the primary effect of fructose and increases lipogenesis, and in the case of diet soft drinks, by the additional contribution of aspartame sweetener and caramel colorant which are rich in advanced glycation end products that potential increase insulin resistance and inflammation."

Soft drinks consumption and nonalcoholic fatty liver disease.
Nseir W. Et al. World J Gastroenterol. 2010 Jun 7;16(21):2579–88.

✦

"We found that 80% of patients with non-alcoholic fatty liver disease had excessive intake of soft drink beverages compared to 17% of healthy controls. The most common soft drinks were Coca-Cola (regular, 32%; diet, 21%) followed by fruit juices (47%)."

Soft drink consumption is associated with fatty liver disease independent of metabolic syndrome. Abid A, et al. J Hepatol. 2009 Nov;51(5):918–24.

✦

"Consumption of fructose in patients with non-alcoholic fatty liver disease was nearly 2- to 3- fold higher than controls. The pathogenic mechanism underlying the development of NAFLD may be associated with excessive dietary fructose consumption."

Fructose consumption as a risk factor for non-alcoholic fatty liver disease. Ouyang X, et al. J Hepatol. 2008 Jun;48(6):993–9.

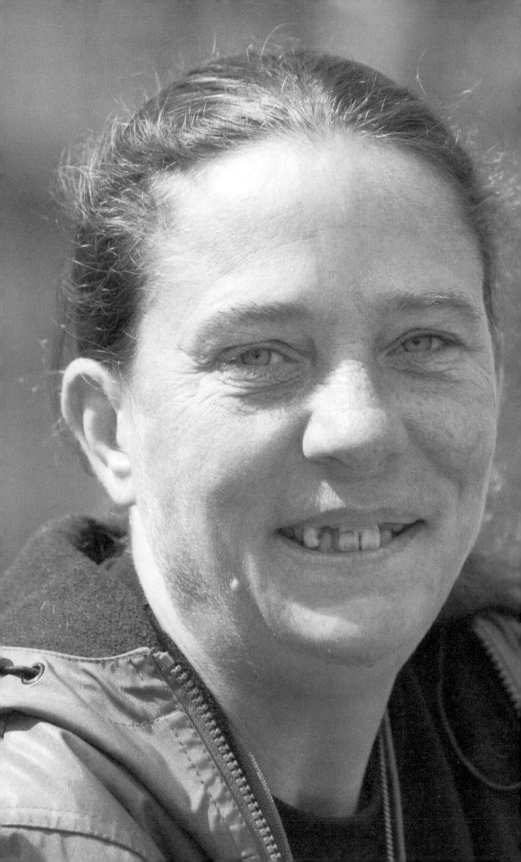

Chapter Nine

Oral Hygiene's
Sweet Disaster

I t was a long time coming but finally, in 2014, a prominent medical journal published the definitive scientific study telling consumers what many of us had already had intuitively known: eating sugar triggers not just tooth decay, but initiates the more serious condition called periodontal disease, a gum impairment which leads to even more devastating ailments.

Writing in the *American Journal of Clinical Nutrition*, a team of five scientists described how they studied data from 2,437 young adults, ages 18 to 25, and estimated their sugar intake using food-frequency questionnaires. Periodontal disease in the study participants was considered to be present based on gum bleeding on probing to a depth of about 3 mm at one or more gum sites.

In both the upper and middle levels of sugar consumption among the young adults, periodontal disease was found. The sugar connection was clear.[79]

It's known that the type of bacteria producing periodontal disease thrive when the human mouth is an acidic environment, which is what dietary sugars are expert at creating. When those bacteria and resultant plaque produce inflammation of the gums around the teeth, gingivitis starts and if left untreated, evolves into pyorrhea, a chronic degenerative gum condition resulting in tooth loss.

Periodontal disease is accelerated even more as a result of nutritional deficiencies, such as Vitamin C and Vitamin D deficits. These deficiencies also destroy bone around the teeth and the periodontal ligaments anchoring your teeth to your jawbone.

It's estimated that up to 75% of all American adults, and most likely the same in most developed countries, currently have some degree of gum disease, mostly as a result of high sweetener usage.[80]

In postmenopausal women, it's well established that the loss of bone density, the disease commonly called osteoporosis, can be traced in part to the occurrence of periodontal disease. One reason is that periodontal conditions can combine with postmenopausal estrogen deficiencies to dramatically reduce bone mineral density. Whole Food Vitamin and mineral supplements are important for these women to take in order to help correct the risk factors.

Among other findings in the sugar consumption=periodontal disease=other ailments scenario is the connection to Rheumatoid arthritis. (See more about this connection in the next chapter, Chapter 10, on sugars and bone and muscle health.)

Still another connection exists between sugar consumption, periodontal disease, and the onset and severity of diabetes.

After reviewing research on the common links between sugar, periodontal disease, and diabetes, Dr. Steven W. Seibert, an Illinois specialist in the field of Periodontology, noted how the sugar link swings both ways: "Research has emerged that suggests that the relationship between periodontal disease and diabetes goes both ways. Periodontal disease may make it more difficult for people who have diabetes to control their blood sugar, and people who have uncontrolled diabetes and uncontrolled blood sugar level may be more prone to having periodontal disease."[81]

We've come a long way in our understanding of sugar's toxic effects on the human mouth since 1983, when a report in the British medical journal, *The Lancet*, observed: "Sugar is the principal cause of the most common disease in industrialized countries, dental caries (decay)."

Now with confirmation that sweeteners are directly linked to periodontal disease and not just tooth decay, medical science can finally begin to explore all of the many possible ways that migration of toxic bacteria from the mouth, caused by sugar consumption, can wreak havoc on the human body and its health.

Study Evidence Overview for Sugar Causing Tooth Decay

"Interviews were carried out by trained fieldworkers who asked about dental health. A total of 1,700 interviews were carried out. Of the children aged 3–17 years, 56% had received treatment for decay (fillings or teeth removed due to decay). Intake of non-milk extrinsic sugars increased the risk of having had treatment for decay. The raised risk remained in children who reported brushing their teeth at least twice a day."

Sugar intake and dental decay: results from a national survey of children in Scotland. Masson LF, et al. Br J Nutr. 2010 Jul 19;1–10.

✦

"A cross sectional study of 165 children aged 3 to 11 years was undertaken to investigate the relationship between diet and severe tooth decay. The children had between 1 and 20 decayed missing or filled primary teeth; 37% ate a chocolate bar daily, and 29% regularly drank a sugary drink after brushing their teeth."

Dietary and Social Characteristics of Children with Severe Tooth Decay. Cameron FL. Et al. Scottish Medical Journal. 2006 August;51(3):26–29.

✦

"Diet affects the integrity of the teeth: quantity, pH, and composition of the saliva; and plaque pH. Sugars and other fermentable carbohydrates, after being hydrolyzed by salivary amylase, provide substrate for the actions of oral bacteria, which in turn lower plaque and salivary pH. The resultant action is the beginning of tooth demineralization. Consumed sugars are naturally occurring or are added."

Sugars and dental caries. Touger-Decker R. van Loveren C. Am J Clin Nutr. 2003 October;78(4);8815–8925.

✦

"Sugar is the principal cause of the most common disease in industrialized countries, dental caries. The sugars implicated in dental caries, in decreasing order of cariogenicity, are sucrose, glucose, and fructose; brown sugars are as cariogenic as white. The level of sugar consumption at which most of the population will not get dental caries is 15 kg/person a year. The goal should therefore be to reduce consumption to this level and below."

Sugars and Dental Decay. Sheiham A. The Lancet. 1983 February;321(8319):282–284.

Periodontal Disease and Rheumatoid Arthritis Link

"Periodontal disease is one of the most common chronic disorders of infectious origin known in humans with a prevalence of 10 to 60% in adults. Rheumatoid arthritis and periodontal disease have shown similar physiopathologic mechanisms such as chronic inflammation with adjacent bone resorption. It has been suggested that oral microorganisms, especially periodontal bacteria, could be the infectious agent. There is no question that Rheumatoid arthritis and periodontal disease have pathologic features in common and there is strong evidence of an association between both diseases."

Rheumatoid arthritis and the role of oral bacteria. Loyola-Rodriguez JP. Et al. J Oral Microbiol. 2010;2:10.

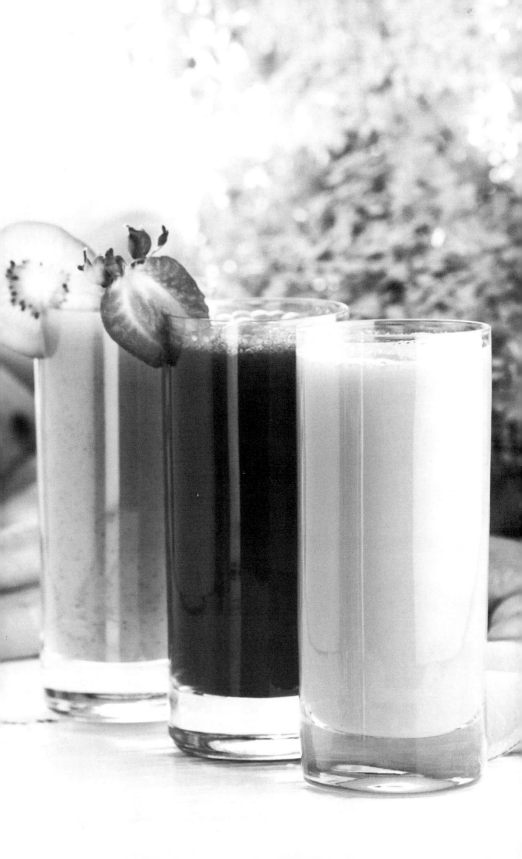

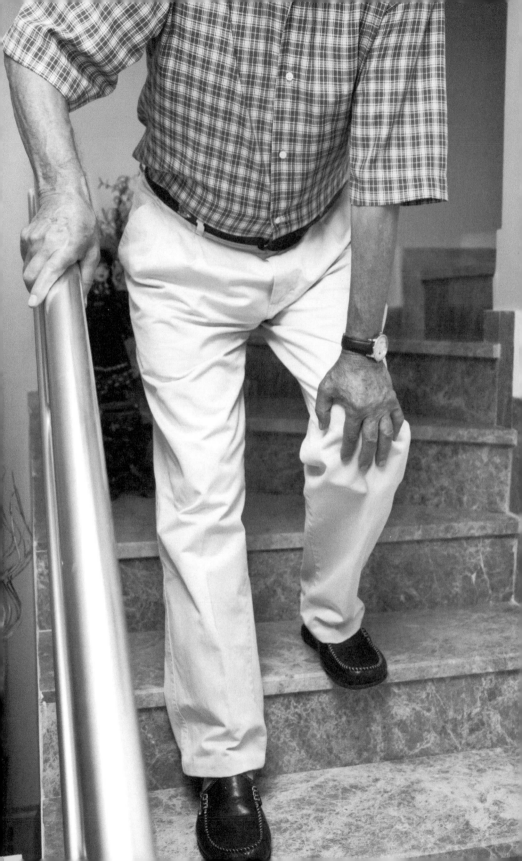

Chapter Ten

Bones and Muscles Deteriorate From Sugar

Sugar and related sweeteners change the chemistry of the human body to such an extent that one of the impacts is to trigger autoimmune diseases that erode cartilage, tissue and bones.

As discussed in the previous chapter, there is a direct connection between Rheumatoid arthritis (RA) and periodontal disease caused by sugar consumption. RA is a chronic inflammatory disorder, an autoimmune disease, and usually attacks the small joints of the feet and hands; the pain experienced is particularly severe in women. For people who contract it, their immune system has been provoked to literally attack itself via cartilage in joints.

But the connection between sugar and related sweeteners and Rheumatoid arthritis is even more direct. You don't necessarily need oral bacteria in the mix.

Scientists writing in the American Journal of Clinical Nutrition examined health data on 186,000 women, evaluating their sugar-sweetened soda consumption, and uncovered a pattern in which "regular consumption of sugar-sweetened soda is associated with increased risk of Rheumatoid arthritis in women, independent of other dietary and lifestyle factors." This 2014 study found the association between sugar intake and RA to be particularly clear in women who were 55 years and older.[82]

Bone quality and bone strength is another body area where sugar wreaks widespread havoc.

Experiments with lab animals have demonstrated a clear pattern—dietary sucrose diminishes bone strength leading to fractures. In the *Journal of Nutrition,* scientists reported that after just five weeks of sucrose consumption, lab animals lost strength in their tibias and femurs. That was true in both males and females, though the breaking point from sucrose was more pronounced in females.[83]

To test whether glucose had more of a negative impact on bone mass and bone strength than fructose, a team of researchers writing in the medical journal, *Bone,* in 2008, fed lab animals both sucrose and fructose sweetened beverages. The experiment lasted eight weeks.

Though both glucose and fructose had a negative impact on bone strength and bone mineral density, it was glucose which "exerted more deleterious effects on mineral balance and bone."[84]

Finally, last but not least, there is gout.

It's a complex form of arthritis, according to The Mayo Clinic, and it can affect anyone, though it is more prevalent in men and afflicts women more often after menopause.[85]

In case you've never experienced it, gout shows up suddenly, often with searing, burning pain in the joint of the big toe. The affected joint is hot to the touch, swollen and tender.

Gout attacks are caused by a build-up of uric acid, which in turn results from eating certain foods high in a substance called purines, such as steak, seafood, and alcoholic beverages.

Sugars are one of the culprits in triggering gout attacks.

Both dietary fructose and sucrose consumption have been identified in studies as contributing to the uric acid build-up in the bloodstream, triggering gout. Sugar-sweetened beverages, including fruit juices, are a primary source for contaminating the body with fructose and sucrose.

"With each extra daily sugar-sweetened beverage serving, a 15% increase in risk" for gout occurred, reported the medical journal, *Annals of Rheumatoid Disease*, in 2014.[86, 87]

More Study Evidence on
Sweeteners and Bone Strength

"The objective of this study was to determine the effect of drinking different sugar-sweetened beverages on bone mass and strength. The results suggested that glucose rather than fructose exerted more deleterious effects on mineral balance and bone."

The effect of feeding different sugar-sweetened beverages to growing female Sprague-Dawley rats on bone mass and strength. Tsanzi E, et al. Bone. 2008 May;42(5):960–8.

Sweeteners and Gout

"Consumption of high fructose corn syrup-sweetened beverages increases serum urate and risk of incident gout. Participants were 1634 New Zealand (European Caucasian). We tested association between sugar (sucrose)-sweetened beverage consumption and prevalent gout. The interaction data suggest that genetic variants in SLC2A9-mediated renal uric acid excretion is physiologically influenced by intake of simple sugars derived from sugar sweetened beverages, increasing gout risk."

Sugar-sweetened beverage consumption: a risk factor for prevalent gout with SLC2A9 genotype-specific effects on serum urate and risk of gout. Batt C. Et al. Ann Rheum Dis. 2014 Dec;73(12):2101–6.

✦

The dietary intake of fructose-rich sugar-sweetened beverages has a significant role in raising serum uric acid levels as well as the risk of contracting gout and cardiovascular disease risk factors.

Effects on uric acid, body mass index and blood pressure in adolescents of consuming beverages sweetened with high-fructose corn syrup. Lin WT, et al. Int J Obes. 2012 Aug 14 {Epub ahead of print}

✦

"Many concerns about the health hazards of calorie-sweetened beverages, including soft drinks and fruit drinks and the fructose they provide, have been voiced over the past 10 years. These concerns are related to higher energy intake, risk of obesity, risk of diabetes, risk of cardiovascular disease, risk of gout in men, and risk of metabolic syndrome. Fructose appears to be responsible for most of the metabolic risks, including high production of lipids, increased thermogenesis, and higher blood pressure associated with sugar or high fructose corn syrup. Some claim that sugar is natural, but natural does not assure safety."

Fructose: pure, white, and deadly? Fructose, by any other name, is a health hazard. Bray GA. J Diabetes Sci Technol. 2010 Jul 1:4(4):1003–7.

FRUCTOSE refined sugar
· white refined sugar
· fruit sugar

Sugar-produced oral bacteria and Rheumatoid Arthritis

"We prospectively followed 79,570 women from the Nurses' Health Study (1980–2008) and 107,330 women from the NHS II (1991–2009). Information on sugar-sweetened soda consumption was obtained from a validated food-frequency questionnaire at baseline and approximately every 4 years during follow-up. Incident Rheumatoid Arthritis cases were validated by medical record review. Regular consumption of sugar-sweetened soda is associated with increased risk of seropositive Rheumatoid Arthritis in women independent of other dietary and lifestyle factors."

Sugar-sweetened soda consumption and risk of developing rheumatoid arthritis in women. Hu Y. Et al. Am J Clin Nutr. 2014 Sep;100(3):959–67.

✦

"Periodontal disease is one of the most common chronic disorders of infectious origin known in humans with a prevalence of 10-60% in adults. Rheumatoid arthritis and periodontal disease have shown similar physiopathologic mechanisms such as chronic inflammation with adjacent bone resoprtion. It has been suggested that oral microorganisms, especially periodontal bacteria, could be the infectious agent. There is no question that Rheumatoid arthritis and periodontal disease have pathologic features in common and there is strong evidence of an association between both diseases."

Rheumatoid arthritis and the role of oral bacteria. Loyola-Rodriguez JP. Et al. J Oral Microbiol. 2010;2:10.

✦

"In recent years, remarkable epidemiological and pathological relationships between periodontal diseases and rheumatic diseases, especially rheumatoid arthritis, have been presented. In this review, we discuss in detail the fact that oral bacterial infections and inflammation seem to be linked directly to the etipathogenesis of rheumatoid arthritis."

The association between rheumatoid arthritis and periodontal disease. Detert J. Et al. Arthritis Research & Therapy. 2010;12:218.

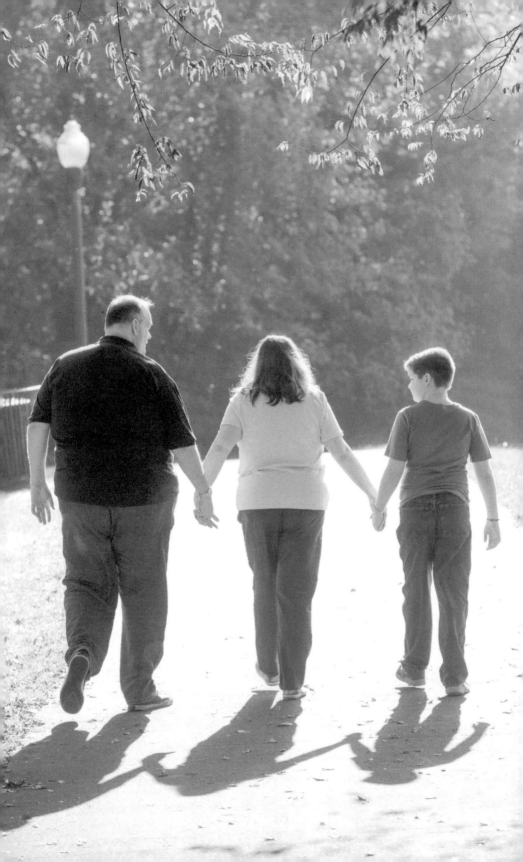

Chapter Eleven

It's Not Just That Sugar Makes You Fat

Sugar consumption initiates a chain reaction of abnormal changes within the human body.

To begin with, added sugars accumulate within your body over time to upset the balance of hormones that maintain many important bodily functions. Glucose levels rise in the bloodstream and that causes your pancreas to release more insulin.

At the next stage, this new infusion of insulin causes your body to store more calories as fat. Excess insulin also unbalances your leptin levels, the hormone that tells your brain that you are full and can quit eating now.

Since your brain can no longer hear the normal stop eating signals, more weight gain occurs and with it comes obesity. With obesity comes sluggishness and insufficient physical exercise, which brings on more weight gain.

A vicious cycle has begun and obesity sets in motion its own chain reaction of unhealthy changes within your body.

Your waist size expands with obesity, your cholesterol and blood pressure usually go up, so do your triglyceride and blood sugar levels. The result is a condition known as Metabolic Syndrome, a cluster of symptoms and abnormalities that greatly increase your risk for contracting diabetes, heart disease, liver disease, and having a stroke.

"Over time, consuming large quantities of added sugar can stress and damage critical organs, including the pancreas and liver," commented scientists at the group Sugar Science, explaining how eating sugar can lead to Metabolic Syndrome. "When the pancreas, which produces insulin to process sugars, becomes overworked, it can fail to regulate blood sugar properly. Large doses of the sugar fructose also can overwhelm the liver, which metabolizes fructose. In the process, the liver will convert excess fructose to fat, which is stored in the liver and also released into the bloodstream."

Five Symptoms Together Equal Metabolic Syndrome

1) **Large waist size:** 40 inches or more for men, 35 inches or more for women.

   is a type of fat

2) **High triglyceride levels:** 150 mg/dL or higher.

3) **Abnormal total cholesterol, or HDL levels:** under 40 mg for men, 50 mg for women.

4) **High blood pressure:** 135/85 mm or higher.

5) **Abnormal blood sugar:** 100 mg/dL or higher.[88]

How many people in the U.S. have been afflicted with metabolic syndrome?

Nearly one in five Americans over the age of 20 has a diagnosable case of it, according to the American Heart Association. Europe, Australia, New Zealand, Canada and all of Western Europe all show similar statistics.

That's enough victims for us to call it what it is—an epidemic.

More Study Evidence on
Sugars and Obesity

"We provide our opinion and review of the data to date that we need to reconsider consumption of dietary sugar based on the growing concern of obesity and type 2 diabetes. Meta-analyses suggest that consumption of sugar-sweetened beverages is related to the risk of diabetes, the metabolic syndrome, and cardiovascular disease. Randomized controlled trials in children and adults lasting 6 months to 2 years have shown that lowering the intake of soft drinks reduced weight gain."

Dietary sugar and body weight: have we reached a crisis in the epidemic of obesity and diabetes? Health be damned! Pour on the sugar. Bray GA. Popkin BM. Diabetes Care. 2014 Apr;37(4):950–6.

✦

"In this review, we evaluate whether there is sufficient scientific evidence that decreasing sugar-sweetened (SSB) beverage consumption will reduce the prevalence of obesity and its related diseases. Findings from well-powered prospective cohorts have consistently shown a significant association and demonstrated a direct-dose response relationship between SSB consumption and long-term weight gain and risk of type 2 diabetes. A meta-analysis of cohort studies also found that higher intake of SSB's among children was associated with 55% higher risk of being overweight or obese compared to those with lower intake. Another meta-analysis of eight prospective cohort studies found that one to two servings per day of SSB intake was associated with a 26% greater risk of developing type 2 diabetes compared with occasional intake (less than one serving per month.)

Resolved: there is sufficient scientific evidence that decreasing sugar-sweetened beverage consumption will reduce the prevalence of obesity and obesity-related diseases. Hu FB. Obes Rev. 2013 Aug;14(8):606–19.

✦

"The consumption of sucrose-sweetened soft drinks has been associated with obesity, the metabolic syndrome, and cardiovascular disorders in observational and short-term intervention studies. We compared the effects of sucrose-sweetened soft drinks with those of isocaloric milk and a noncaloric soft drink on changes in total fat mass and ectopic fat disposition in liver and muscle tissue. Daily intake of sucrose-sweetened soft drinks for 6 months increases ectopic fat accumulation and lipids and is likely to enhance the risk of cardiovascular and metabolic diseases."

Sucrose-sweetened beverages increase fat storage in the liver, muscle, and visceral fat depot: a 6-mo randomized intervention study. Maersk M, et al. Am J Clin Nutr. 2012 Feb;95(2):283–9.

✦

Sugar-sweetened beverages include the full spectrum of soft drinks, fruit drinks, energy and vitamin water drinks, are composed of sucrose, high fructose corn syrup, or fruit juice concentrates. These "promote weight gain and contribute to increased risk of type 2 diabetes and cardiovascular risk factors."

Sweeteners and Risk of Obesity and Type 2 Diabetes: The Role of Sugar-Sweetened Beverages. Malik VS, Hu FB. Curr Diab Rep. 2012 Jan 31 {Epub ahead of print}

✦

"A cross-sectional study was conducted in Tehran, Iran, with 460 women aged 20-50 y. Dietary intake in the previous year was collected by a semi-quantitative food frequency questionnaire. Our data showed that a dietary pattern high in processed meats, soft drinks, sweets, refined grains, snacks and processed juice might be positively associated with obesity."

The association of general and central obesity with major dietary patterns of adult women living in Tehran, Iran. Rezazadeh A, Rashidkhani B. J Nutr Sci Vitaminol (Tokyo) 2010;56(2):132–8.

✦

"In a meta-analysis of the relationship between soft drink consumption and cardiometabolic risk, there was a 24% overall increased risk comparing the top and bottom quantiles of consumption. Fructose acutely increases thermogenesis, trigylcerides and lipogenesis as well as blood pressure. The present review concludes on the basis of the data assembled here that in the amounts currently consumed, fructose is hazardous to the cardiometabolic health of many children, adolescents and adults."

Soft drink consumption and obesity: it is all about fructose.
Bray GA. Curr Opin Lipidol. 2010 Feb;21(1):51–7.

✦

"Sugar-sweetened beverages (SSBs) are beverages that contain added caloric sweeteners such as sucrose, high-fructose corn syrup or fruit-juice concentrates, all of which result in similar metabolic effects. They include the full spectrum of soft drinks, carbonated soft drinks, fruitades, fruit drinks, sports drinks, energy and vitamin water drinks, sweetened iced tea, cordial, squashes and lemonade, which collectively are the largest contributor to added sugar intake in the US. Only recently have large epidemiological studies been able to quantify the relationship between SSB consumption and long-term weight gain, type 2 diabetes and cardiovascular disease risk. Experimental studies have provided important insight into potential underlying biological mechanisms. It is thought that SSBs contribute to weight gain in part by incomplete compensation for energy of subsequent meals following intake of liquid calories. They may also increase risk of type 2 diabetes and cardiovascular disease as a contributor to a high dietary glycemic load leading to inflammation, insulin resistance and impaired beta-cell function. Additional metabolic effects from the fructose fraction of these beverages may also promote accumulation of visceral adiposity, and increased hepatic de novo lipogenesis, and hypertension due to hyperuricemia. Consumption of SSBs should therefore be replaced by healthy alternatives such as water, to reduce risk of obesity and chronic diseases."

Sugar-sweetened beverages and risk of obesity and type 2 diabetes: epidemiologic evidence. Hu FB, Malik VS. Physiol Behav. 2010 Apr 26;100(1):47–54.

◆

"High-fructose corn syrup accounts for as much as 40% of caloric sweeteners used in the United States. The current study examined both short and long-term effect of HFCS on body weight, body fat, and circulating triglycerides. Over the course of 6 or 7 months, both male and female rats with access to HFCS gained significantly more body weight than control groups, accompanied by an increase in adipose fat, notably in the abdominal region, and elevated circulating triglyceride levels. Translated to humans, these results suggest that excessive consumption of HFCS may contribute to the incidence of obesity."

High-fructose corn syrup causes characteristics of obesity in rats: Increased body weight, body fat and triglyceride levels. Bocarsly ME, et al. Pharmacol Biochem Behav. 2010 Feb 26 {Epub ahead of print}.

✦

"Soft drink consumption is now considered to be a major public health concern with implications for cardiovascular diseases. This follows a number of studies performed in animals suggesting that chronic consumption of refined sugars can contribute to metabolic and cardiovascular dysregulation. In particular, the monosaccharide fructose has been attracting increasing attention as the more harmful sugar component in terms of weight gain and metabolic disturbances. High-fructose corn syrup is gradually replacing sucrose as the main sweetener in soft drinks and has been blamed as a potential contributor to the current high prevalence of obesity. There is also considerable evidence that fructose, rather than glucose, is the more damaging sugar component in terms of cardiovascular risk."

Sugary drinks in the pathogenesis of obesity and cardiovascular diseases. Brown CM, et al. Int J Obes (Lond). 2008 Dec;32 Suppl 6:S28–34.

✦

"The odds ratio of becoming obese among
children increases 1.6 times for each additional can
or glass of sugar-sweetened drink consumed beyond
their usual daily intake of the beverage. Soft drinks
currently constitute the leading source of added
sugars in the diet and exceed the U.S. Department of
Agriculture's recommended total sugar consumption
for adolescents."

*The role of sugar-sweetened beverage consumption in adolescent
obesity: a review of the literature.* Harrington S. J Sch Nurs.
2008 Feb;24(1):3–12.

✦

"Consumption of sugar-sweetened beverages,
particularly carbonated soft drinks, may be a key
contributor to the epidemic of overweight and obesity
by virtue of these beverages' high added sugar content.
We reviewed 30 publications selected on the basis of
relevance and quality of design and methods. Their
findings show a positive association between greater
intakes of sugar-sweetened beverages and weight gain
and obesity in both children and adults."

*Intake of sugar-sweetened beverages and weight gain:
a systematic review.* Malik VS, et al. Am J Clin Nutr.
2006 Aug;84(2):274–88.

✦

"Carbohydrates with high glycemic indexes and high glycemic loads produce substantial increases in blood glucose and insulin levels after ingestion. The continued intake of high-glycemic-load meals is associated with an increased risk of chronic diseases such as obesity, cardiovascular disease, and diabetes."

Low-glycemic-load diets: impact on obesity and chronic diseases. Bell SJ, Sears B. Crit Rev Food Sci Nutr. 2003;43(4):357–77.

✦

"Overweight subjects who consumed fairly large amounts of sucrose (28% of energy), mostly as beverages, had increased energy intake, body weight, fat mass, and blood pressure after 10 wk. These effects were not observed in a similar group of subjects who consumed artificial sweeteners."

Sucrose compared with artificial sweeteners: different effects on ad libitum food intake and body weight after 10 wk of supplementation in overweight subjects. Raben A, et al. Am J Clin Nutr. 2002 Oct;76(4):721–9.

Sugar and Metabolic syndrome

"Metabolic syndrome can be caused by modification of diet by means of {the}consumption of high carbohydrate and high fat diet such as fructose. We conclude that the metabolic syndrome rat model is best established with the induction of fructose drinking water for eight weeks. This was evident in the form of higher obesity parameter which caused the development of metabolic syndrome."

The establishment of metabolic syndrome model by induction of fructose drinking water in male Wistar rats. Mamikutty N. Et al. Biomed Res Int. 2014 June 18. {Epub ahead of print}

✦

"The consumption of sucrose-sweetened soft drinks has been associated with obesity, the metabolic syndrome, and cardiovascular disorders in observational and short-term intervention studies. We compared the effects of sucrose-sweetened soft drinks with those of isocaloric milk and a noncaloric soft drink on changes in total fat mass and ectopic fat disposition in liver and muscle tissue. Daily intake of sucrose-sweetened soft drinks for 6 months increases ectopic fat accumulation and lipids and is likely to enhance the risk of cardiovascular and metabolic diseases."

Sucrose-sweetened beverages increase fat storage in the liver, muscle, and visceral fat depot: a 6-mo randomized intervention study. Maersk M, et al. Am J Clin Nutr. 2012 Feb;95(2):283–9.

✦

"We conclude that even moderate consumption of
fructose-containing liquids may lead to the onset of
unfavorable changes in the plasma lipid profile and
one marker of liver health, independent of significant
effects of sweetener consumption in body weight."

*Effect of moderate intake of sweeteners on metabolic health in the
rat.* Figlewicz DP, et al. Physiol Behav. 2009 Dec 7;98(5):618–24.

✦

"High sweetened beverage consumption is
independently associated with the prevalence
of metabolic syndrome in specific sex-ethnicity
populations."

*Comparison of dietary intakes associated with metabolic syndrome
risk factors in young adults: the Bogalusa Heart Study.* Yoo S, et al.
Am J Clin Nutr. 2004 Oct;80(4):841–8.

✦

"The feeding of sugars as compared to starch
produced undesirable changes in metabolic risk factors
such as blood triglycerides, total cholesterol and its
lipoprotein distribution, insulin and uric acid. Other
dietary components (e.g., saturated fat) can magnify
the adverse metabolic effects of the sugars."

*Effect of dietary sugars on metabolic risk factors associated with
heart disease.* Reiser S. Nutr Health. 1985;3(4):203–16.

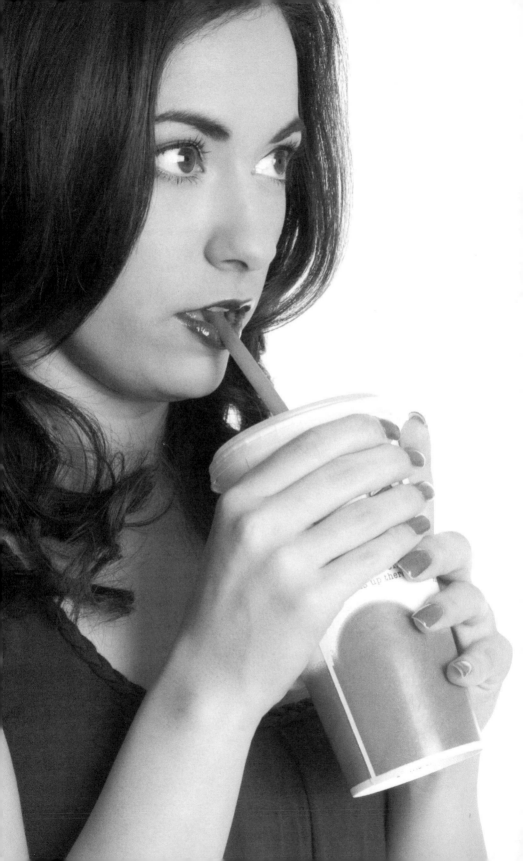

Chapter Twelve

Artificial Sweeteners Are a Bad Substitute

W hen sales of Diet Pepsi began falling in 2005, and continued to fall each year since, PepsiCo executives frantically tried to find out why. The reason turned out to be that consumers had heard about health problems associated with aspartame, the sweetener added to Diet Pepsi, and they no longer trusted it or wanted it in their bodies.

Sold under such names as Equal and NutraSweet, aspartame had been extensively studied, with research both supporting and disputing its safety in humans. Health conditions implicated in the use of aspartame ranged from headaches and depression to memory loss, weight gain and obesity, even neurological problems and cancer.

Enough doubt about its health impact surfaced that on a Twitter sentiment scale of 0 to 100, with Christmas ranked at 88 and the U.S. Congress ranked at 38, aspartame got a lowly 22 ranking, according to the industry tracker *Beverage Digest.*

So the soft drink manufacturer decided in April 2015 to replace aspartame in Diet Pepsi with sucralose, another artificial sweetener better known as Splenda. This chlorinated sugar is a substance with almost as many health question marks as the sweetener it replaced.

For example, a team of scientists in Israel tested the entire range of non-caloric artificial sweeteners, including sucralose, saccharin and aspartame, on lab animals. They used doses corresponding to the acceptable daily intake in humans set by the U.S. Food and Drug Administration. They also did follow-up experiments using human volunteers to confirm the animal findings.

They published their findings in an October 2014 issue of the science journal, *Nature,* concluding that the more artificial sweeteners used the greater the bacterial growth associated with type 2 diabetes. Other markers for diabetes—raised blood sugar levels and glucose intolerance—were also induced by artificial sweeteners used in a group of 381 human volunteers.[89]

"Our findings suggest that non-caloric artificial sweeteners may have directly contributed to enhancing the exact epidemic {obesity} that they themselves were intended to fight," commented Eran Segal, a study co-author with the Weizmann Institute of Science.

The scientists speculated that absorbing artificial sweeteners expands the numbers of a bacterial species living in the intestines that store energy as fat, leading to obesity and as a consequence, type 2 diabetes. It may also be that the sweeteners suppress the growth of other important types of bacteria involved with preventing insulin resistance.

Rather than alleviate obesity-related metabolic conditions, as artificial sweeteners were intended to do by replacing sugar in soft drinks and a range of processed food products, these chemicals actually contribute to developing those very health problems by tinkering with the balance of healthy and unhealthy bacteria in the gut. The food industry and soft drink manufacturers just substituted one health undermining evil for another.

"Artificial sweeteners, which are present in high doses in diet soda, are associated with a greater activation of reward centers in the brain, thus altering the reward a person experiences from sweet tastes," observed a 2014 report by the Johns Hopkins Bloomberg School of Public Health. "In other words, among people who drink diet soda, the brain's sweet sensors may no longer provide a reliable gauge of energy consumption because the artificial sweetener disrupts appetite control. As a result, consumption of diet drinks may result in increased food intake overall."[90]

As more recent evidence indicates, it gets even worse!

Researchers at the University of Iowa Hospitals and Clinics used health data from nearly 60,000 participants (post-menopausal women) in the Women's Health Initiative to determine the impact of all artificial sweeteners on heart health. Writing in an April 2015 issue of the *Journal of General Internal Medicine*, the 10 scientists involved in the study found a clear link between soft drink intake and cardiovascular disease and resultant death among post-menopausal women.[91]

Those women who consumed two or more diet drinks a day were 30% more likely to experience a cardiovascular event (heart attack or stroke) and 50% more likely to die from cardiovascular disease compared to women who didn't consume diet drinks containing artificial sweeteners.

These studies are just the beginning of a continuing cycle of intensive research into the role that artificial sweeteners play in triggering health problems.

"Synthetic chemical sweeteners are generally unsafe for human consumption," warned Dr. James Bowen, who has studied these substances for two decades after he found that aspartame triggered his Lou Gehrig's disease. "Don't be deceived. These chemicals are toxic."[92]

15
CALORIES
PER SERVING

Splenda
BRAND SWEETENER®

™

Nutriti
Serving Size
Servings Per

Amount Per Ser

Calories 15

Total Fat 0g

Sodium 10mg

Total Carbohydra

Sugars 3g

Protein 0g

Vitamin C 100%

Not a significant
in fat, saturated
dietary fiber

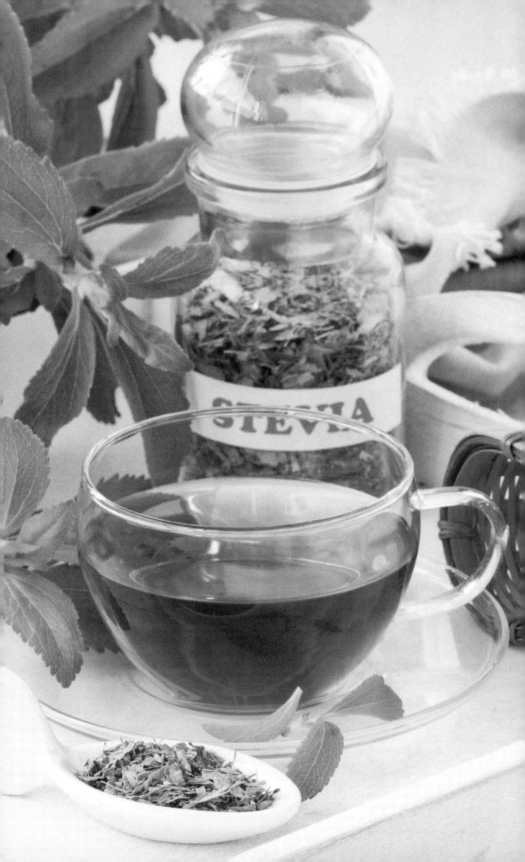

Appendix One:
A Safe Sweetener
Alternative—Stevia

I t's extracted directly from a plant, it's up to 200 times sweeter than table sugar, it contains no calories, and it doesn't come with the health problems associated with other sweeteners.

We're talking about stevia, a South American plant that has been used by indigenous peoples for hundreds of years to make tea and sweeten beverages. They also historically used it for its medicinal properties to treat stomach upset.

Though the word 'stevia' is associated with the entire plant, the components of it which are sweet have the technical name of 'steviol glycosides' and come from the leaves of the plant.

The medical journal *Appetite* featured a study in 2010 showing the effects of sugar, stevia, and artificial sweeteners in a group of experimental subjects. Stevia had by far the fewest health complications and after consuming it, study participants had lower blood sugar and lower insulin levels overall than those who consumed sugar or aspartame.

There is even study evidence that stevia lowers blood pressure in hypertension patients and can be useful in the treatment and management of diabetes.

No adverse reactions to its use have been documented, so stevia has been labeled safe to use by most of the world's health organizations.

It's sold under a variety of names and labels including, but not limited to, PureVia, Stevioside, Stevia Extract in The Raw, SweetLeaf, Steviacane, Enliten, or just plain Stevia.

Though the sugar and artificial sweetener industries tried for decades to suppress the sale and use of stevia, mostly by concocting phony claims about safety, it has gradually become a fixture in consumer buying choices.

As consumers have discovered, stevia can effectively substitute for sugar, aspartame and other artificial sweeteners in a wide range of edible goods: desserts, sauces, pickled foods, chewing gum, prepared vegetables, etc.

Science Evidence for
Stevia Safety and Healing Properties

"We studied the effects of stevia leaves and its extracted polyphenols and fiber on diabetic rats. We hypothesize that supplementation of polyphenols extract from stevia in the diet causes a reduction in diabetes and its complications. The results suggested that stevia leaves do have a significant role in alleviating liver and kidney damage in diabetic rats, besides the hypoglycemic effect."

Antioxidant, anti-diabetic and renal protective properties of Stevia rebaudiana. Shivanna N. Et al. J Diabetes Complications. 2013 Mar-Apr;27(2):103–13.

✦

"The safety of steviol glycoside {stevia} sweeteners has been extensively reviewed in the literature. National and international food safety agencies and approximately 20 expert panels have concluded that steviol glycosides, including the widely used sweeteners stevioside and rebaudioside A, are not genotoxic. This review establishes the safety of all steviol glycosides with respect to their genotoxic/carcinogenic potential."

Steviol glycosides safety: is the genotoxicity database sufficient? Urban JD. Et al. Food Chem Toxicol. 2013 Jan;51:386–90.

✦

"Our results {tested in diabetic rats} support the validity of an extract of Stevia rebaudiana leaves for the management of diabetes as well as diabetes-induced renal disorders."

Effects of Stevia rebaudiana (Bertoni) extract and N-nitro-L-arginine on renal function and ultrastructure of kidney cells in experimental type 2 Diabetes. Ozbayer C. Et al. J Med Food. 2011 Oct;14(10):1215–22.

✦

"This review serves as a clinical support tool. Evaluation of two long-term studies (1 and 2 years in length) indicates that stevia may be effective in lowering blood pressure in hypertensive patients. A pair of small studies also report positive results with respect to glucose tolerance and response."

An evidence-based systematic review of stevia by the Natural Standard Research Collaboration. Ulbricht C. Et al. Cardiovasc Hematol Agents Med Chem. 2010 Apr;8(2):113–27.

Appendix Two:
Recipes to Please Without Sickness

W e are honored to present sugar-free recipes prepared by two of our talented raw food chefs at the Hippocrates Health Institute.

Ken Blue is the Executive Chef of the Hippocrates kitchen whose culinary training began as a child working and playing at his grandfather's restaurant. After graduating from Emory University with a degree in Biology, he opened a vegetarian restaurant. He became Executive Chef at Hippocrates in 2005. In addition to preparing cuisine for our guests and leading raw cooking classes, Ken offers monthly classes on living food preparation for the general public as well as overseeing the culinary portion of our Health Educator Program.

Renate Wallner was born in the beautiful southern alps of Austria and for the past decade has worked in the Hippocrates kitchen learning and perfecting the art of making raw food dishes without sugar. She has also focused on developing and teaching simple sugar free raw food menus for "entertaining at home." Look for her book on sugar free entertaining in the near future.

No honey mustard

Ingredients:

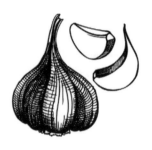

2½ ounces lemon juice

1 garlic cloves

½ tsp kelp powder

¾ tbsp. yellow mustard

10 drops stevia

1 tbsp turmeric

2 cups parsnips, small cut

6 ounces sesame oil

Directions:

In a blender, add all the ingredients and blend until smooth. Add water-a little bit at a time, about ½ cup, to adjust consistency, if necessary.

Almost 1000 Island

Ingredients:

5 ounces fresh lemon juice

3 garlic cloves

1½ tsp kelp powder

Pinch of cayenne

2 red bell pepper, roughly cut, divided

1½ large parsnip, cut into small pieces

¾ cup extra virgin olive oil

Water if necessary to adjust consistency

To blend in a food processor:

3 cucumbers, sliced

2 white onions, chopped

2 small bottles of capers, without the liquid

Directions:

In a blender mix all the ingredients until smooth.

Fold in the mixture from the food processor until combined. Refrigerate.

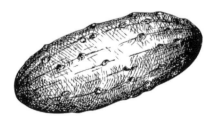

Dijonnaise

Ingredients:

1 clove of garlic

5 ounces fresh lemon juice

5 tbsp brown mustard seeds

3½ cups parsnip, small cut

1 tbsp dried thyme

1 tsp kelp

1¼ cups sesame oil

Water, if necessary to adjust consistency

Directions:

In a blender add all ingredients and process until smooth.
Adjust consistency adding water a little bit at a time, if needed.

Sugar Free Holiday Nog

Ingredients:

1 cup almonds, soaked overnight

1 cup sunflower seeds, or pine nuts, soaked overnight

4 cups of water

½ teaspoon ground nutmeg

½ teaspoon cinnamon

4 drops Stevia, or more to taste

2 tablespoon vanilla flavor, without alcohol

Directions:

In a blender, prepare the milks separately as follows:

For almond milk: Blend 1 cup of almonds with 2 cups of water. Pour and squeeze through nut milk bag.

For sunflower/pine nuts milk: Blend 1 cup sunflower seeds or pine nuts with 2 cups of water. Pour and squeeze through a nut milk bag.

Add milks, stevia, vanilla, nutmeg, and cinnamon in a blender. Blend well. Serve or refrigerate for up to 2 days.

Sweetheart Salad

Ingredients:

1 Butternut Squash, Peeled & Seeded

1 Sweet Potato

1 Carrot

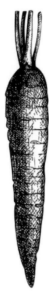

Dressing:

¾ C. Chopped Carrot

⅛ C. Lemon Juice

½ C. Raw, Organic Sesame Oil

¾ Tsp. Ginger, Minced

¾ Tsp. Kelp Powder

1 Tsp. Cinnamon

¾ Tsp. Pumpkin Pie Spice

½ Tiny Scoop Stevia Powder

1 Tbsp. Frontier Vanilla (without alcohol)

Directions:

1. In a food processor, thinly slice squash, sweet potato and carrot.

2. In a strong blender, blend dressing to smooth consistency.

3. Toss and serve.

Cinnamon cookies

YIELD 15 COOKIES

Ingredients:

2 cups pecans, soaked overnight and rinsed
¼ teaspoon Stevia
1 tablespoon cinnamon
1 tablespoon vanilla flavor, without alcohol
Pinch of nutmeg
Water, if needed to adjust consistency

Directions:

Drain and rinse the pecans and put in a food processor with cinnamon, stevia, vanilla, and nutmeg.

Process until pecans have been fully ground and the mixture begins to form a ball.

Take small amounts of the mixture and form with your hands into cookies.

Lay into a dehydrator tray.

Dehydrate at 105°F overnight.

Serve warm to family and friends.

Red Pepper Ketchup

Ingredients:

2 C. Chopped Red Bell Pepper

2 Tsp. Garlic Powder

¼ C. Chopped Red Onion

1 Pinch Ground Clove

⅛ C. Chopped Red Beet   *sugar*

⅔ C. Extra Virgin Olive Oil

2 T. Paprika

1½ T. Fresh Lemon Juice

2 T. Ground Flax Seed

¼ Tsp. Liquid Stevia Extract

1 T. Celery Powder*(or 1 stalk of celery)

Directions:

1. In a blender, combine all ingredients.
2. Blend well and season to taste.

Celery powder is made by dehydrating celery, then grinding it to a powder using a spice grinder or dry blender.

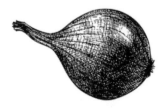

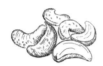

Nut or Seed Milk

Nut Milk:

Soak any type of nut or seed
overnight & rinse
(discard water)

Blend 2 C soaked and rinsed nuts
or seeds with 5 C. water on
high speed for 20 seconds

Squeeze through sprout bag

Nut Milk will stay fresh in the refrigerator for up to 3 days.

Flavorings can be included once the pulp is removed if desired.

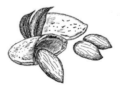

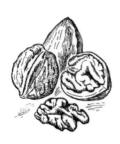

Nut Ice Cream

3 quarts nut milk
(equal parts walnuts & pine nuts)

To make nut milk for ice cream:

Soak nuts overnight & rinse
(discard water)

Blend 2 cups walnuts & 2 cups water

Squeeze through sprout bag

Blend 2 cups pine nuts & 2 cups water

Squeeze through sprout bag

Alternate this process between walnuts and pine nuts until
there is 3 quarts of nut milk (nut "cream")

Add to nut milk:

4 oz vanilla flavor (alcohol free)

4 T cinnamon

1 oz Frontier maple flavor

2 capfuls stevia

(To adjust sweetness, add either more vanilla or stevia)

Lastly, follow the directions on your ice cream maker.

Chia Pudding

Ingredients:

¼ C. Chia Seed

1 C. Brazil Nut Milk

Vanilla Bean

Unsweetened Shredded Coconut

Directions:

1. Add Brazil nut milk to the chia seed.
2. Let it sit for 15 min and stir intermittently.
3. Add more nut milk as needed to desired texture.

Optional: add vanilla and unsweetened shredded coconut.

*To make Brazil nut milk, blend 2 C. brazil nuts (soaked overnight and rinsed thoroughly) and 5 C. of water on high speed for 20 seconds. Squeeze through a sprout/nutmilk bag.

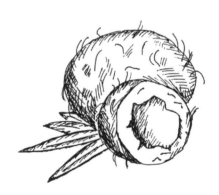

Very veggie dressing

Ingredients:

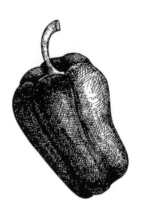

2½ ounces lemon juice

1½ cloves of garlic

½ red pepper, coarsely chopped

½ carrot, sliced

½ green zucchini, roughly cut

½ yellow squash, roughly cut

½ teaspoon kelp

2 tablespoons pizza seasoning

5 ounces extra virgin olive oil

Directions:

Blend all the ingredients in a blender until smooth. Adjust consistency, if necessary, adding water while the blender is running.

Note: The sweetness of the vegetables in this dressing makes it sweet enough. However, you can always add Stevia if needed.

Ken's Almost Shortbread Cookies

YIELD 45 COOKIES

Ingredients:

3 Cups Brazil nuts,
soaked overnight and rinsed

3¾–4 Cups of sliced carrots

¼ tsp cinnamon

2 tsp vanilla flavor, without alcohol

18 drops Stevia

Zest of 1 lemon

2 ounces fresh lemon juice

Method:

In a large bowl, mix all ingredients. Run the combined ingredients through a juicer using a blank screen.

Combine all again. Spread mix, about a ¼ inch thick, over a paraflex sheet and place sheet on top of a dehydrator tray.

Dehydrate on the sheet for the first day at 110°F. Then the next day, dehydrate off the sheet at the same temperature.

If by the third day the cookies are thoroughly dehydrated, take off the sheet and place in a sealed container. They will last for a month or two.

Sugar-free Lemonade

SERVE 1

Ingredients:

8 oz water

2.5 ml (1½ tsp.) fresh lemon juice

8 drops stevia

1 slice lemon

1 slice lime

Directions:

Pour water in a glass. Add fresh lemon juice and stevia. Lightly squeeze slices of lemon and lime and add to the water. Mix well to combine. Drink.

Sugar-Free Chai Latte

YIELD 1

Ingredients:

1 Tbsp roobois tea

½ tsp tsp garam masala

⅛ tsp cinnamon

¼ tsp nutmeg

8 oz homemade almond milk

1 drop stevia

Instructions:

Combine roobois tea and spices. Make tea. Add almond milk and stevia. Stir to combine well. Serve hot or cold.

This mix contains no black pepper.

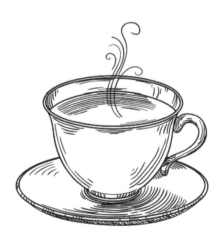

Red Pepper Tahini Dressing

Ingredients:

2 + ½ Red Bell Peppers, Roughly Chopped

2 oz. Lemon Juice

1 + ½ cloves garlic

1 + ½ TBSP Frontier Pizza Seasoning

7 Drops Stevia

¼ tsp Kelp Powder

7 oz. Raw Organic Tahini

Directions:

1. In a blender, combine all ingredients, except Tahini.

2. Blend well, then add Tahini and Blend again.

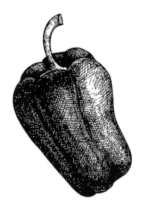

Following recipes by: Renate Wallner
Sugar Free Raw Vegan Cuisine

Holiday Pumpkin Pie

YIELD 1 8-INCH PIE

Ingredients:

For the filling:

3 cups pumpkin, thinly sliced

2 cups carrots, thinly sliced

1½ cups of water

¼ tbsp. pumpkin spice

½ tbsp. cinnamon

2 tbsp vanilla, alcohol free

½ tsp stevia

1 tbsp psyllium

For the crust:

3 cups of pecans, soaked, rinsed and dehydrated

1 tbsp cinnamon

1 tbsp mesquite powder

1 tbsp vanilla

Directions:

To make the filling:

Add all ingredients except the psyllium in a blender and process until smooth.

Add in the psyllium and blend well.

To make the crust:

Add all ingredients in a food processor and process until well combined.

Place mixture in an 8-inch pie mold pan, press down using your hands to form the crust. Add the filling on top and refrigerate.

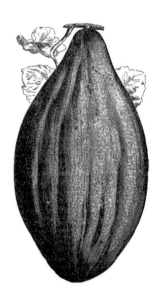

Walnut Truffle/Blondies

Chop in food processor until fine:

3½ cups soaked & dehydrated walnuts then add:

1 T vanilla, ½ t stevia and 1 T water

Process and pulse until mixture forms a ball

(Do not over process)

Press mixture into a flat dish for Blondies or roll into bite size truffles.

For variation roll truffles in shredded coconut or shopped dehydrated nuts.

Refrigerate or serve as is. Truffles will keep in refrigerator for 8 weeks.

Vanilla Cream Topping

Blend until smooth:

1 cup nut milk

1 cup soaked macadamia nuts

1 t lemon juice, 1 T liquid vanilla, alcohol free

¼ t stevia, pinch of sea salt

After blending above well, add:

1 t lecithin,

¼ cup coconut oil (soft/melted)

blend until well incorporated

Vanilla cream will keep in refrigerator for 5 days

Coconut Cheese Cake

Crust:

Chop very fine in food processor:

3 cups dehydrated pecans

Then add:

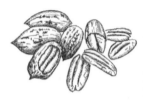

1 T vanilla (alcohol free), ¼ t stevia, 1 T water

Process until it holds together and press into cake form

Filling:

Blend until thick and creamy:

2 cups macadamia nuts (soaked)

1 cup shredded dried coconut

1½ cups almond milk

1 cup coconut water

¾ t stevia and 3 T liquid vanilla, alcohol free

blend until smooth

Stop blending and add:

3 T lecithin powder and 1 cup coconut oil/melted

now blend on medium until well incorporated

Pour this creamy filling into the crust.

Freeze for 3 hours until firm, then keep cake in the refrigerator.

Cake will keep in fridge for 5 days

Creamy Cole Slaw

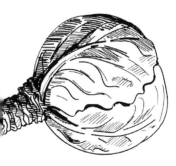

Ingredients:

4 cups thinly sliced
green cabbage

½ cup thinly sliced
red cabbage

½ cup shredded carrots

Dressing:

Blend until very creamy

¼ cup lemon juice

1 clove garlic

1 t celery seeds

½ t mustard powder

3 cups parsnips, chopped

1 cup sesame oil

¾ cup water

5 drops stevia, optional

Toss everything together in a large mixing bowl.
This makes a wonderful picnic salad.

References

Introduction: An Unsweet Story, an Unhappy Ending

1 Ng SW. Et al. *Use of Caloric and noncaloric sweeteners in US consumer packaged foods*. J Acad Nutr Diet. Nov. 2012;112(11):1828–34.

2 "Sugar Season. It's Everywhere, and Addictive." James J. DiNicolantonio, Sean C. Lucan. The New York Times. Dec. 22, 2014.

3 "Panel Calls for Less Sugar and Eases Cholesterol Restrictions." The New York Times. Feb. 20, 2015. A13.

4 "The growing concern over too much added sugar in our diets." Sugar Science, University of California at San Francisco. *www.sugarscience. org*

5 "Where is added sugar hiding?" Sanjay Gupta. CNN. March 10, 2015. *http://www.cnn.com/videos/tv/2015/03/10/orig-added-sugar-sanjay-gupta-calories-food.cnn*

6 *Dietary sugar and salt represent real risk factors for cataract development*. Veromann S. Et al. Opthalmologica. 2003 Jul–Aug;217(4):302–7.

7 *Associations of Western and traditional diets with depression and anxiety in women*. Jacka FN. Et al.Am J Psychiatry. 2010 Mar;167(3):305–11.

8 *Sugary soda consumption and albuminuria: results from the National Health and Nutrition Examination Survey, 1999–2004*. Shoham DA. Et al. PLoS One. 2008;3(10):e3431.

9 Sugar Association v. Corn Refiners Association. History of the case, 2013. Online at *http://sweetsurprise.com/western-sugar-litigation-case-history*.

10 International Food Information Council Foundation. 2012. Sugars and health resource page. *http://www.foodinsight.org/Resources/Detail.aspx?topic=Sugars_and_Health_Resource_Page*.

11 Comments by General Mills on the National School Lunch and School Breakfast Programs: Nutrition Standards for All Foods Sold in School. Document FNS-2011-0019. Comment ID FNS-2011-0019-3716. Food and Nutrition Service, USDA.

12 "Added Sugar, Subtracted Science: How Industry Obscures Science and Undermines Public Health Policy on Sugar." June 2014. Center for Science and Democracy. *www.ucsusa.org/addedsugar*.

13 Brown, D.A. *Ethical analysis of disinformation campaign's tactics.* 2012. Penn State Rock Ethics Institute.

14 "Coke A Good Snack? Health Experts Who Work With Coke Say So." Associated Press. March 16, 2015.

15 *www.robynflipse.com*

16 "Sugar-Sweetened Beverages." *www.sugarscience.org*.

17 *Consumption of added sugars and development of metabolic syndromes components among a sample of youth at risk of obesity.* Wang, J. Applied Physiology, Nutrition, and Metabolism. 2014 April;39(4):512.

18 "The hidden costs of sugar." November 14, 2014. *http://medicalxpress.com/print335173008.html*

Chapter One: Sugar's Notorious History—A Timeline

19 "A Brief History of Honey." The Honey Association. *http://www.honeyassociation.com/index.asp?pid=9*

20 *A Splendid Exchange: How Trade Shaped the World.* William Bernstein. 2009. London: Atlantic Books.

21 "Adult Obesity Facts." Centers for Disease Control and Prevention. *http://www.cdc.gov/obesity/data/adult.html*

22 Alzheimer's Foundation of America. Statistics. *http://www.alzfdn.org/AboutAlzheimers/statistics.html*

23 "Cancer Statistics." NIH Fact Sheets. National Institutes of Health. *http://report.nih.gov/nihfactsheets/viewfactsheet.aspx?csid=75*

24 "Cancer Trends During the 20th Century." Journal of Australian College of Nutritional & Environmental Medicine. Vol. 21, No. 1. April 2002.

25 "Diabetes Public Health Resource." Centers for Disease Control and Prevention. *http://www.cdc.gov/diabetes/statistics/prev/national/figby age.htm*

26 *Dietary sugars intake and cardiovascular health: A scientific statement from the American Heart Association.* Circulation, 120:1011–1020.

27 "History of Type 2 Diabetes." Healthline. April, 2013. *http://www. healthline.com/health-slideshow/history-type-2-diabetes#3*

28 "How Sugar is Made—the History." *http://www.sucrose.com/lhist. html*

29 "Is sugar the missing link in RA? Weissmann G. Internal Medicine News. 2006;39(16):11.

30 "Major Milestones in Alzheimer's Research." Alzheimer's Association. *http://www.alz.org/research/science/major_milestones_in_alzheimers. asp*

31 "Periodontitis Health Guide." The New York Times. *http://www. nytimes.com/health/guides/disease/periodontitis/risk-factors.html*

32 "Processed Food: A 2-Million-Year History." *Scientific American.* Vol. 309, Issue 3. *http://www.scientificamerican.com/article/processed -food-a-two-million-year-history/*

33 "Sugar Consumption in the US Diet between 1822 and 2005." Guyenet, Stephan & Landen, Jeremy. Online Statistics, Rice University and Tufts University. *http://onlinestatbook.com/2/case_studies/sugar.html*

34 "Sugar Love." Rich Cohen. National Geographic. August, 2013.

35 "Sugar and Sweeteners." Anderson J. & Young L. Colorado State University, Fact Sheet No. 9.301. Food and Nutrition Series. Revised May 2010.

36 "The Real Bad Egg Is Sugar." *The New York Times.* Feb. 19, 2015.

37 *The Sugar Barons: Family, Corruption, Empire and War.* Matthew Parker. 2011. London: Hutchinson.

38 "Why Did Thematoid Arthritis Begin in 1800?" Richard S. Panush, M.D. *The Rheumatologist.* Sept. 2012. *http://www.the-rheumatologist. org/details/article/2543901/Why_Did_Rheumatoid_Arthritis_Begin_ in_1800.html*

Chapter Two: Our Most Addictive Substance

39 *Intense sweetness surpasses cocaine reward.* Lenoir M. Et al. PLoS One. 2007 Aug 1;2(8):e698.

40 Sugar can be addictive, Princeton scientist says. Princeton University. Dec. 10, 2008. *http://www.princeton.edu/main/news/archive/ S22/88/56G31/index.xml?section=topstories*

41 "Rats treat Oreos like cocaine, study suggests." Eoin O'Carroll. The Christian Science Monitor. Oct. 16, 2013.

42 *Animal models of sugar and fat bingeing: relationship to food addiction and increased body weight.* Avena NM. Et al. Methods Mol Biol. 2012;829:351–65.

43 *Sweet preference, sugar addiction and the familial history of alcohol dependence: shared neural pathways and genes.* Fortuna JL. J Psychoactive Drugs. 2010 Jun;42(2):147–51.

44 *Sugar addiction: pushing the drug-sugar analogy to the limit.* SH Ahmed. Et al. Curr Opin Clin Nutr Metab Care. 2013 Jul;16(4):434–9.

45 *If sugar is addictive…what does it mean for the law?* Gearhardt A. Et. al. J Law Med ethis. 2013 Mar;41 Suppl 1:46–9.

46 *The Origins of Fruits, Fruit Growing, and Fruit Breeding.* Janick, J. Plant Breeding Review. 2005. 25:255–330.

47 Janick; pg. 56–60.

48 "Breeding the Nutrition Out of Our Food." Jo Robinson. *The New York Times.* May 25, 2013.

49 Action on Smoking and Health. "Tobacco Additives: Cigarette Engineering and Nicotine Addiction." *http://www.ash.org.uk/files/docu ments/ASH_623.pdf*

50 *Breaking the Food Seduction*. Neal Barnard. 2003, St. Martin's Press.

Chapter Three: Cancer Cells Get Addicted to Sugar, Too

51 Does cancer love sugar? *http://www.mdanderson.org/patient-and-cancer-information/cancer-information/cancer-topics/prevention-and-screening/food/cancersugar.html*

52 "Does Sugar Feed Cancer?" ScienceDaily. August 18, 2009. *http://www.sciencedaily.com/releases/2009/08/090817184539.htm*.

53 *Refined fructose and cancer*. Liu H. Heaney AP. Expert Opin Ther Targets. 2011 Sep; 15(9):1049–59.

54 *Fructose consumption and cancer: is there a connection?* Port AM. Et al. Curr Opin Endocrinol Obes. 2012 Oct;19(5):367–74.

55 *Dietary patterns and risk of mortality from cardiovascular disease, cancer, and all causes in a prospective cohort of women*. Heidemann C, Et al. Circulation. 2008 Jul 15;118(3):230–7.

56 (American Cancer Society, Cancer Statistics, 2013: *http://onlinelibrary.wiley.com/doi/10.3322/caac.21166/full*)

Chapter Four: Diabetes Has a Sugar Connection

57 "It's the Sugar, Folks." Mark Bittman. *The New York Times*. February 27, 2013.

58 *The relationship of sugar to population-level diabetes prevalence: an econometric analysis of repeated cross-sectional data*. Basu S, Yoffe P, Hills N, Lustig RH. PLoS One. 2013;8(2):e57873.

59 *Added Fructose: A Principal Driver of Type 2 Diabetes Mellitus and Its Consequences*. DiNicolantonio JJ. Et al. Mayo Clin Proc. 2015 Jan. 26: S0025–6196(15)00040–3.

60 *Consumption patterns of sugar-sweetened beverages in the United States*. Han E. Powell LM. J Acad Nutr Diet. 2013 Jan;113 (1):43–53.

61 *Daily sugar-sweetened beverage consumption and insulin resistance in European adolescents: the HELENA (Healthy Lifestyle in Europe by Nutrition in Adolescence Study*. Kondaki K. Et al. Public Health Nutr. 2013 Mar;16(3):479–86.

62 *Association between sugar-sweetened and artificially sweetened soft drinks and type 2 diabetes: systematic review and dose-response meta-analysis of prospective studies.* Greenwood DC. Et al. Br J Nutr. 2014 Sep 14;112(5):725–34.

63 *Resolved: there is sufficient scientific evidence that decreasing sugar-sweetened beverage consumption will reduce the prevalence of obesity and obesity-related diseases.* Hu FB. Obes Rev. 2013 Aug;14(8):606–19.

64 "Alcohol and Blood Sugar." The Global Diabetes Community. www.diabetes.co.uk/alcohol-and-blood-sugar.html.

65 "Hidden levels of sugar in alcohol revealed." Edward Malnick. *The Telegraph* (UK). March 29, 2014.

Chapter Five: Heart attacks, cardiovascular disease, hypertension, stroke—the sugar connection

66 "Sugar Kills! How Do We Decrease Consumption?" J. Ritterman. *The Huffington Post*. March 20, 2014.

67 *Added Sugar intake and cardiovascular disease mortality among US adults.* Yang Q. Et al. JAMA Internal Medicine. 2014 April; 174(4):516–524.

68 "Eating too much added sugar increases the risk of dying with heart disease." Julie Corliss. *The Harvard Heart Letter*. Feb. 6, 2014.

Chapter Six: Your Brain on Sugar Equals Alzheimer's, Depression, Cognitive, Memory and Behavioral Problems

69 *Hippocampal apoptosis involved in learning deficits in the offspring exposed to maternal high sucrose diets.* Kuang H. Et al. J Nutr Biochem. 2014 Sep;25(9):985–90.

70 *The effect of beverages varying in glycaemic load on postprandial glucose responses, appetite and cognition in 10–12 year old school children.* Brindal E. Et al. Br J Nutr. 2013 Aug 28;110(3):529–37.

71 *http://www.nlm.nih.gov/medlineplus/ency/article/002426.htm*

72 *Cinnamon counteracts the negative effects of a high fat/high fructose diet on behavior, brain insulin signaling and Alzheimer-associated changes.* Anderson RA. Et al. PLoS One. 2013 Dec 13;8(2):e83243.

Chapter Seven: Sugars Accelerate Your Aging

73 *Does dietary sugar and fat influence longevity?* Archer VE. Med Hypotheses. 2003 Jun;60(6):924–9.

74 *Soda and cell aging: associations between sugar-sweetened beverage consumption and leukocyte telomere length in healthy adults from the National Health and Nutrition Examination Surveys.* Leung CW. Et al. Am J Public Health. 2014 Dec;104(12):2425–31.

75 *High serum glucose levels are associated with a higher perceived age.* Noordam R. Et al.Age. 2013 Feb;35(1):189–95.

Chapter Eight: Non-Alcoholic Fatty Liver Disease from Sweeteners

76 *Pediatric Nonalcoholic Fatty Liver Disease: A comprehensive Review.* Lindback SM. Et al. Advances in Pediatrics. 2010;57(1):85–140.

77 *The Epidemiology of Nonalcoholic Fatty Liver Disease: A Global Perspective.* Lazo M. Et al. Seminars in Liver Disease. 2008;28(4):339–50.

78 *Adipose tissue as an endocrine organ.* Kershaw EE. Et al. The Journal of Clinical Endocrinology and Metabolism. 2004 June;89(6):2548–56.

Chapter Nine: Oral Hygiene's Sweet Disaster

79 *Added sugars and periodontal disease in young adults: an analysis of NHANES III data.* Lula EC. Et al. Am J Clin Nutr. 2014 Oct;100(4):1182–7.

80 "Gum Disease Overview." *The New York Times. www.nytimes.com/ health/guides/disease/periodontitis/risk-factors.*

81 "Elevated sugar and gum disease." *http://www.gumdoc.net/periodontal -diseases/blood-sugar.html*

Chapter Ten: Bones and Muscles Deteriorate From Sugar

82 *Sugar-sweetened soda consumption and risk of developing rheumatoid arthritis in women.* Hu Y. Et al. Am J Clin Nutr. 2014 Sept;100(3):959–67.

83 *A high-sucrose diet decreases the mechanical strength of bones in growing rats.* Larmas M. Et al. J Nutr. 1998 Oct;128(10):1807–10.

84 *The effect of feeding different sugar-sweetened beverages to growing female Sprague-Dawley rats on bone mass and strength.* Tsanzi E. Et al. Bone. 2008 May;42(5):960–8.

85 *http://www.mayoclinic.org/diseases-conditions/gout/basics/definition/con-20019400*

86 *Sugar-sweetened beverage consumption: a risk factor for prevalent gout with SLC2A9 genotype-specific effects on serum urate and risk of gout.* Batt C. Et al. Ann Rheum Dis. 2014 Dec;73(12):2101–6.

87 *Sugar-sweetened beverages, urate, gout and genetic interaction.* Merriman TR. Pac Health Dialog. 2014 Mar;20(1):31–8.

Chapter Eleven: It's Not Just That Sugar Makes You Fat

88 "Making Sense of Metabolic Syndrome." *http://www.sugarscience.org/*

Chapter Twelve: Artificial Sweeteners Are a Bad Substitute

89 *Artificial sweeteners induce glucose intolerance by altering the gut microbiota.* Korem T. Et al. Nature. Oct. 9, 2014.

90 *Diet Beverages Are Not the Solution for Weight Loss.* Johns Hopkins Bloomberg School of Public Health. January 16, 2014. *http://www.jhsph.edu/news-releases/2014/diet-beverages-not-the-solution-for-weight-loss*

91 *Diet drink consumption and the risk of cardiovascular events: a report from the Women's Health Initiative.* Vyas A. Et al. J Gen Intern Med. 2015 Apr;30(4):462–8.

92 "The Lethal Science of Splenda, A Poisonous Chlorocarbon." James Bowen, M.D. May 8, 2005. *http://www.holisticmed.com/splenda/bowen.html*

About The Author

Brian Clement has directed Hippocrates Health Institute now in West Palm Beach, Florida since 1980. This internationally renowned health center has been helping people to help themselves since 1956. More than 400,000 people from over 70 countries have been guests in the Life Transformation Program and thousands more have become certified Hippocrates Health Educators. Clement and the Institute have spearheaded major trends in the field of natural health care over the decades.

As a licensed PhD nutritionist who has training as a nautropathic doctor and has worked in nutrition for the last four decades, he possesses priviledged insight into what is required to regain and maintain health. His focus in this book is on the devasting effect of all forms of sugar relating to human health. This is one of his foremost concerns, and he hopes to put an end to its abuse.

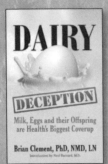
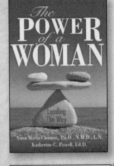
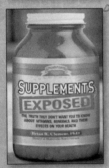
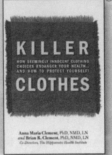
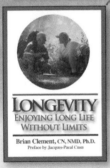
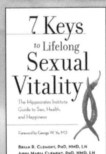
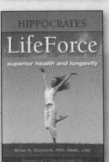
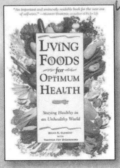

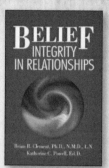

Belief: Integrity in Relationships
by Brian Clement, PhD, LN and Katherine Powell, EdD

Belief offers a blueprint for helping people attain health in body, mind, emotion, and relationships.

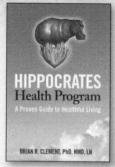

Hippocrates Health Program
by Brian Clement, PhD, LN

Brian Clement has been a leader in the health field for over three decades. He directs Hippocrates Health Institute in South Florida, which promotes sane living in a polluted, stressful and undernourished world.

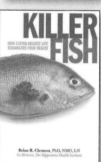

Killer Fish
by Brian Clement, PhD, LN

People the world over are eating more fish than ever before and assuming fish to be a healthful alternative to meat as well as an excellent source for omega-3 fatty acids. *Killer Fish* alerts consumers to how eating aquatic life endangers their health.

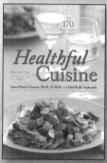

Healthful Cuisine
by Anna Maria Clement, PhD, LN & Kelly Serbonich

If you're one of the millions of people who have learned about the superior health and nutritional benefits of raw and living foods and want to begin experiencing its life-enhancing qualities, then Healthful Cuisine is for you!

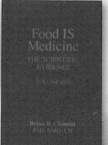

Food IS Medicine: Volume One
THE SCIENTIFIC EVIDENCE
by Brian Clement, PhD, LN

Book one in a three-volume series presenting data from studies clearly demonstrating that the most important ingested medicine comes from the food we consume.

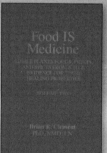

Food is Medicine: Volume Two
EDIBLE PLANT FOODS, FRUITS, AND SPICES FROM A TO Z
by Brian Clement, PhD, LN

Book two in a three-volume series presenting data from studies clearly demonstrating that the most important ingested medicine comes from the food we consume.

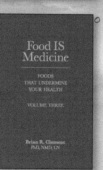

Food is Medicine: Volume Three
FOODS THAT UNDERMINE YOUR HEALTH
by Brian Clement, PhD, LN

Book three in a three-volume series presenting data from studies clearly demonstrating that the most important ingested medicine comes from the food we consume.